Getting a PhD in Health and Social Care

withdrawn
17/6/22

Immy Holloway *PhD, MA, BEd, CertEd*

Jan Walker *PhD, BSc, RGN, RM, RHV, CPsychol*

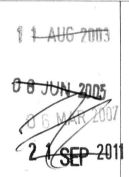

Blackwell Science

Don Gresswell Ltd., London, N.21   Cat. No. 1207

DG 02242/71

© 2000 by
Blackwell Science Ltd
Editorial Offices:
Osney Mead, Oxford OX2 0EL
25 John Street, London WC1N 2BL
23 Ainslie Place, Edinburgh EH3 6AJ
350 Main Street, Malden
  MA 02148 5018, USA
54 University Street, Carlton
  Victoria 3053, Australia
10, rue Casimir Delavigne
  75006 Paris, France

Other Editorial Offices:

Blackwell Wissenschafts-Verlag GmbH
Kurfürstendamm 57
10707 Berlin, Germany

Blackwell Science KK
MG Kodenmacho Building
7–10 Kodenmacho Nihombashi
Chuo-ku, Tokyo 104, Japan

The right of the Author to be identified as
the Author of this Work has been asserted
in accordance with the Copyright, Designs
and Patents Act 1988

First published 2000

Set in 10.5/13 pt Sabon
by Aarontype Limited, Easton, Bristol
Printed and bound in Great Britain by
MPG Books Ltd, Bodmin, Cornwall

The Blackwell Science logo is a
trade mark of Blackwell Science Ltd,
registered at the United Kingdom
Trade Marks Registry

DISTRIBUTORS

Marston Book Services Ltd
PO Box 269
Abingdon
Oxon OX14 4YN
(*Orders*: Tel: 01235 465500
            Fax: 01235 465555)

USA
Blackwell Science, Inc.
Commerce Place
350 Main Street
Malden, MA 02148 5018
(*Orders*: Tel: 800 759 6102
                    781 388 8250
            Fax: 781 388 8255)

Canada
Login Brothers Book Company
324 Saulteaux Crescent
Winnipeg, Manitoba R3J 3T2
(*Orders*: Tel: 204 837 2987
            Fax: 204 837 3116)

Australia
Blackwell Science Pty Ltd
54 University Street
Carlton, Victoria 3053
(*Orders*: Tel: 03 9347 0300
            Fax: 03 9347 5001)

A catalogue record for this title
is available from the British Library

ISBN 0-632-05057-8

Library of Congress
Cataloging-in-Publication Data

Holloway, Immy.
    Getting a Phd in health and social
    care/Immy Holloway, Jan Walker.
        p. cm.
    Includes bibliographical references and
    index.
    ISBN 0-632-05057-8 (pbk.)
    1. Social work educational – Great
Britain. 2. Community heath services –
Study and teaching (Graduate) – Great
Britain. 3. Human services – Research.
4. Dissertations, Academic. I. Walker,
Jan, 1946– . II. Title.
HV11.8.G7H65 1999
361'.0071'141 – dc21   99–35390
                                      CIP

For further information on Blackwell
Science, visit our website:
www.blackwell-science.com

To our supervisors
Bob Colquhoun and Justus Akinsanya

Contents

Foreword

It is a great pleasure to write a foreword to this book by two highly experienced academics. The book is balanced and provides authoritative accounts of key issues in postgraduate studies for the MPhil or PhD.

The use of real-life examples, with their instructive and challenging stance, should make this an important book for all postgraduate researchers. The contents reflect the many problems and challenges which postgraduate researchers face in the quest for completion of their MPhil or PhD. One of the challenges faced by health and social care professionals is how their research base can be developed, nurtured and strengthened. The authors have responded to these issues by providing a book that is authoritative, with its materials arranged in a systematic and logical way.

In 13 chapters, the book deals with relevant and up-to-date research materials. It covers approaches to the development of ideas for study, through to the completion stage. The book begins with a clear discussion of the nature of the research degree, covering such important preliminary issues as part-time and full-time study and choosing between an MPhil or a PhD. It ends appropriately with a robust discussion on dissemination in Chapter 12.

Any textbook such as this which aims to inform and prepare MPhil and PhD postgraduate students for the research process must be applauded. Although the emphasis throughout is necessarily on the MPhil/PhD postgraduate, the materials in the book apply to all researchers and will be invaluable to their quest for research-based qualifications.

For all the above reasons, I highly recommend the book as a reliable guide to all aspects of research for higher degrees, and more especially as a handbook for the practical problems which arise in the course of any type of research. In short, the book is an indispensable aid for researchers and those undertaking health and social care research courses. It should also serve as useful background or reference reading for those involved in promoting research generally.

Professor Justus A. Akinsanya
BSc, PhD, RGN, ONC (Hons), BTA, CertRNT, FRCN, FWACN, FRSH
Emeritus Professor of Nursing Studies
Anglia Polytechnic University, UK

Preface

About this book

Our book is designed to provide advice and practical guidelines for health and social care professionals who study for an MPhil or a PhD.

There has been an increasing interest by those working, or wishing to work, in the field of health and social care in gaining higher academic qualifications. A number of factors have contributed to this, including the move of nurse and midwifery education to higher education; the expansion of degree courses in health, social studies and community care; and increasing numbers of social workers and those in the professions allied to medicine who have graduated. In the last few years, this has led to many more people enrolling in universities to obtain an MPhil or PhD. Most of these are mature students who have been stimulated by academic courses and wish to extend their knowledge and further their careers. Some are young professionals who have achieved good degrees and want to continue academic study. Most, though by no means all, have professional qualifications and study part-time. The rapid rate of their enrolment and registration for research degrees means that, within a few years, numbers will have grown dramatically and will go on increasing.

Studies related to health and social care lie at the interface between established scientific disciplines in the social and biomedical sciences. Most higher degrees will, of necessity, draw on these. Those who study for an MPhil or PhD in these fields come from a variety of academic and practice backgrounds. They will have obtained first degrees in a diverse range of disciplines, such as nursing, one of the social sciences, health sciences, a biological science, education, physiotherapy or chiropractic. Medical practitioners too are increasingly seeking to gain a higher degree in topics related to health and social care, rather than the pure biomedical sciences. Depending on their academic background or subject discipline, those seeking to register for a higher degree in this field may already have substantial expertise in research methods; others have very little knowledge of methods at all.

It is our view that individuals registering for a higher degree in health or social care are likely to encounter a number of common problems which are not necessarily faced by those working in other, 'pure' disciplines. These include the demands of establishing and managing supervisory arrangements for work which crosses disciplinary boundaries; gaining access and working within settings which provide both working and living environments; ethical issues related to dealing with sensitive topics and vulnerable groups; and presenting findings which honestly represent all relevant points of view but, if negative, will not damage the morale of those involved in care provision or prejudice future research opportunities. This is why, in our opinion, there is the need for a book specifically on the process of studying for an MPhil or PhD in the field of health and social care in the UK.

Our text aims to complement the increasing number of excellent general texts on thesis and dissertation writing by providing advice specifically aimed at professionals and others working in this field of study. It focuses particularly on applied research which involves working with people, whether these are patients, clients or fellow professionals.

How to use this book

This book is targeted, in the first instance, at those who are just thinking about the possibility of studying for a higher degree in this field. Part 1 is designed to assist potential students to negotiate their way through the minefield of decisions and bureaucratic processes involved in enrolment and registration. Readers may be surprised at the length of this section, but we believe that attention to details at this stage of the process resolves most of the problems likely to be encountered later on. Part 2 is concerned with the processes involved in achieving a successful MPhil or PhD, following registration. In our experience, professionals from backgrounds relevant to health and social care often lack the confidence and assertiveness to take charge of decisions which can have far-reaching personal and professional effects. This book is intended to enable them to take control over these processes. It also draws attention to some of the issues specifically faced by researchers whose studies involve working in applied settings, in addition to some of the problems common to all research students. Those who do not have a professional background or experience of working in the field may find some of these sections particularly helpful (for example, how to manage 'gatekeepers').

The headings, contents and summaries for each chapter are intended to allow students to 'dip into' topics as they appear relevant. However, we would encourage students to read ahead, as the book is intended primarily to pre-empt possible problems and thus help the reader to avoid some of the most common pitfalls and impediments to success. The list of references and suggestions for further reading are, of course, not comprehensive but aim to assist students to extend their knowledge of research.

The authors

Immy Holloway is a Reader in the Institute of Health and Community Studies, Bournemouth University. She is an educationalist and medical sociologist with a PhD in the field of the sociology of occupations. Jan Walker is a nurse and health psychologist who has held readerships at Bournemouth University and King Alfred's College, Winchester, and is currently principal lecturer in multiprofessional health care at the University of Plymouth. Her PhD focused on pain in elderly people living in the community. Both authors have experience in supervising MPhil and PhD students in nursing and midwifery as well as those from backgrounds in medicine, social work and other professional disciplines. Both have managed the process of postgraduate research student supervision from admission to examination, as well as organising research training and seminar programmes for students and staff in their respective departments and institutions.

Both authors are actively engaged in their own research programmes, and their presentations and publications include issues related to the conduct of research in health and community care. Immy Holloway is the author of the text *Basic Concepts in Qualitative Research* (Blackwell Science, Oxford, 1997) which is written mainly for health professionals, social workers and teachers. She has also co-authored *Qualitative Research for Nurses* (Blackwell Science, Oxford, 1996) with Stephanie Wheeler. Jan Walker is co-author, with Sheila Payne, of *Psychology for Nurses and the Caring Professions* (Open University, Buckingham, 1996) and has also written a number of book chapters on pain in the elderly.

Part 1

Preparation

Chapter 1

The Nature of the Research Degree

The research degree in health and social care

The majority of research in the field of health and social care is applied research. This type of research covers the full range of human experience. Participants may be patients, clients, carers, professionals, students or members of the general public. They include those with physical, mental health or intellectual disabilities; those who are well, those who are sick or dying; those in distress and those who are coping well; those receiving and those giving care; those who make policy, those who manage or implement policy and those who educate. Settings for this type of research include people's own homes, residential homes or institutions, hospitals or hospices, centres of education and even the streets.

Applied research involves the collection and analysis of primary data, and the presentation of findings, which have explicit implications for practice, education or policy. Some research studies will involve the direct testing of interventions in practice, using scientific methods. Others will involve close and detailed observation and/or evaluation of practices and policies using methodologies which do not necessarily fit into traditional scientific approaches.

In contrast, basic research refers to ground-breaking ('blue skies') scientific research which may involve inductive or deductive methods. Such research, for instance, would include the discovery of a genetic structure which, although it has obvious implications for a wide range of applications in health and social care, was not conducted with this primarily in mind. Basic research also refers to theory building and testing which may involve laboratory- or field-based experiments. Again, although theory has obvious implications for the development of interventions and policy-making, its primary purpose is a scientific one.

In spite of the title Master or Doctor of Philosophy, studies in health and social care at this level rarely rely on philosophical methods alone, although some aspect of philosophy will undoubtedly underpin the research approach taken. For example, positivism, social construction- ism, interpretivism and post-modernism are examples of different philo- sophical traditions in which researchers may position themselves and which inform the research methodology used. It is useful to have some basic knowledge of these terms because most research in this field, even that involving traditional scientific methods, depends upon assumptions about the nature of subjective experience and how to deal with different perspectives on reality (for example, one's own, those of professionals and those of clients). For potential research students, not familiar with the importance of these issues, a good introduction can be found in the book by McKenzie *et al*. (1997), referenced at the end of this chapter. It is helpful to discuss and debate these issues with others.

Part-time versus full-time study

Most people have little choice in deciding whether to study full- or part- time. Few people have the luxury, in terms of time or finance, of studying full-time. Those who depend on an income will normally expect to carry on working while they undertake their MPhil or PhD. Indeed, their MPhil or PhD is likely to be closely related to their work. Some of the pros and cons of full-time and part-time study are set out in Fig. 1.1.

The issues raised in Fig. 1.1 speak for themselves in explaining why the suspension and drop-out rate is much higher for part-time than for full-time students. Part-time study requires an extremely high level of time and commitment. Those working in a profession, be it practice related or education based, should reflect carefully on their motives for wishing to obtain a higher degree by research and decide if their aspira- tions are best served by studying for a PhD or an MPhil or, if they do not already have a higher degree, if they would not be better off stud- ying for a taught Masters degree.

Choosing between an MPhil and a PhD

An MPhil denotes an autonomous researcher who demonstrates mastery of all stages of the research process including design, imple- mentation, analysis and writing up. A good reason for studying for an MPhil is to gain competence and confidence in the practical application

Fig. 1.1 Advantages and disadvantages of full-time and part-time study.

Part-time study		Full-time study	
Advantages	Disadvantages	Advantages	Disadvantages
Lower annual fees Career continuity Ready access for applied research Direct opportunities to change practice in response to research findings	Constant interruptions from work and home demands Limited access to academic peer support Prolonged study period can lead to disenchantment Topic may be outdated by completion Time limit constraints Lack of support/ understanding from work colleagues	Full opportunity for intense concentration during working hours Time for enjoyment Full engagement with academic peers and support from research community Regular access to supervisors	Long period out of the job market Isolation from work-related peer group Funding (fees, expenses, subsistence) essential Time limit constraints

of research methods. The MPhil process is a suitable way of acquiring knowledge of research methods, and the MPhil is an appropriate qualification for those wishing to take up a service-based research post and who have the opportunity to engage in their own research or make their own contribution to a larger research programme. It allows the opportunity to carry out a useful piece of field-based research under supervision, while extending knowledge of research methods and their application in practice. Obtaining an MPhil or a taught Masters in social research methods is also an excellent preparation for those working in further or higher education who wish to be research-active and/or teach social research methods. The time commitment required is sufficiently reasonable to enable those working in education or practice to succeed. A successful MPhil thesis (referred to in some institutions as a dissertation) will be of publishable quality, and articles from it are likely to be welcomed by the editors of academic and professional journals.

Those with an MPhil will be able to make a personal contribution to the research and development aspirations of their employers through the writing of research proposals, the design and execution of useful research programmes – in practice, helping others with these activities – and disseminating research findings. Unfortunately, we sense that the MPhil is increasingly, but erroneously, regarded as a failed PhD. In our view, many of those who currently feel under pressure to study for a PhD would be much better advised to aim for an MPhil.

A PhD denotes a researcher who demonstrates all of the attributes associated with the MPhil but has also made a unique contribution to the body of knowledge (through new theoretical or methodological approaches, or new facts) in the chosen field (these issues are discussed further later in this chapter). A doctorate is an important qualification for those who have ambitious career aspirations in higher education, since it provides evidence of academic credibility at the highest level. However, a doctorate is not always advantageous for those wishing to pursue a teaching or service-based career. Those who leave practice or service to study full-time may find it difficult to return as they might be seen as out of date in their practice and possibly too threatening to their seniors or peers. One of us (Jan Walker) found herself in great demand in the NHS after completing her first degree, but virtually unemployable after completing her PhD three years later. The NHS has attempted to address this problem through the provision of studentships which encourage the student to maintain a consultative or practice-based role for about one day per week. However, this can still result in conflict between the demands of work and those of research.

Failure to complete among those attempting to complete a PhD part-time while continuing to work in health or social care is high. Competing work demands, family commitments, new work challenges, changes in work or family circumstances, together with a waning of enthusiasm for the research as the years pass, make it an extremely difficult task.

Registration for MPhil/PhD

Almost all universities now require that students intending to study for a PhD register for MPhil/PhD. Students registering, in the first instance, for an MPhil with the opportunity to transfer to a PhD must demonstrate that they have the ability to study at this level and that their research is likely to fulfil the requirements for the PhD. This provides a safety net for those who, for any reason, do no wish to or are unable to continue and prefer to submit to examination for the MPhil. It also means that those who, in the first instance, decide to opt for an MPhil have the opportunity to progress to a PhD if they subsequently change their mind. Those allowed to register direct for a PhD include students who have successfully completed a research-based Masters course.

Motivations for study at this level

The best reasons for undertaking this type of study are probably: a strong desire to conduct a specific study and, at the same time, demonstrate competence in the research process, in which case an MPhil is probably most appropriate; or a burning motivation to engage in research to learn more about a topic or issue, in which case it is worth aiming for a PhD.

In our experience, some of the best students have been those who have embarked on their journey towards a PhD with a sense of trepidation and uncertainty. One of the worst reasons for undertaking PhD research is to 'prove' a preconceived hypothesis, though students can get away with this for an MPhil if the research is rigorously conducted. Those who seek to demonstrate that a particular approach or intervention is best sometimes fail to acknowledge the existence of alternative arguments or see the relevance of alternative explanations. A biased PhD thesis is a failed thesis.

Some students who have already embarked on, or even conducted, a piece of research in practice wish to have this credited towards a research degree. Very rarely is the work of a suitable standard to contribute to an MPhil, while most PhDs would start by challenging the assumptions on which the work was originally based. Existing research or a sense of missionary zeal can, in some cases, block the desire for further knowledge and prevent the individual from being open to alternative perspectives or ideas. People who believe that they are already experts in their field and deserve a PhD for the work they have already done (but usually never bothered to write up in a readable format) are almost invariably wrong.

It appears to be a truism that the more you learn, the more you realise you don't know. Those who eventually obtain a PhD are usually regarded as experts in a limited field. Most of us who have passed this hurdle realise how much we still have to learn about so many other aspects of our field of study.

The nature of the MPhil

The aim of the MPhil thesis is to demonstrate mastery in the conduct and application of the research process. Someone who has undertaken a good undergraduate dissertation should be able to work in partnership as a valuable member of a research team. Someone who has an MPhil should be able to lead such a research team.

To achieve the award of MPhil, the candidate must demonstrate competence in all aspects of the research process including:

- Formulating the research question(s).
- Writing a research proposal which presents a sound rationale, including an overview of the literature, to support the research aims and chosen methodology.
- Designing and piloting the research study using appropriate methodologies and research instruments.
- Negotiating access and ethical approval.
- Independently conducting or supervising data collection in a rigorous manner.
- Analysing and presenting the data accurately and appropriately.
- Discussing the full implications of the findings, including their validity and reliability.
- Reaching conclusions and recommendations, based on the findings, which directly address the original research issues and question(s).

The MPhil thesis

The MPhil thesis is usually between 40 000 and 60 000 words in length, although theses in the natural sciences may contain less. The number of words varies depending on the requirements of the university concerned. Examination involves the presentation of the thesis and defence in viva voce (oral examination).

The main difference between the undergraduate and the MPhil thesis, apart from length, is that the former emphasises the acquisition of research skills while the latter requires the demonstration of research competence. The MPhil thesis also produces findings which are credible and relevant to practice, and it is of publishable quality.

The nature of the PhD

The emphasis of the PhD is on a process of inquiry or investigation which answers a specific research question or sheds new or significant light on an important issue. The PhD often involves a voyage of discovery through a series of research studies, critical reviews and reflections which combine to contribute to a fresh understanding of the central issue in terms of new theory or different theoretical approaches, new methodologies or different methodological approaches, or new facts.

A typical PhD might involve the following stages:

- Identifying and focusing the central research question.
- Writing the research proposal, identifying preliminary research study and possible developmental work, differentiating between MPhil and PhD outcomes (see Chapter 7 on writing the research proposal).
- Writing a critical review of the existing literature, clearly identifying the need for this PhD research.
- Consideration and justification of the chosen theoretical and/or methodological approach and data collection instruments.
- Designing, piloting, conducting, analysing and writing up the first investigatory study, critically reviewing the process, considering the key findings, and reconsidering the purpose and nature of the next phase.
- During the above phase, students will need to decide whether to continue to a PhD or stop at the MPhil. The transfer or examination procedure, as appropriate, should be initiated at this stage.
- Modifying the research design, as necessary, and conducting the next phase of the PhD investigation, as appropriate.
- Presenting a detailed analysis of the overall findings and their implications.
- Critically reviewing the whole in the light of an updated literature search and review.
- Making recommendations for practice, based on the overall findings.

The doctoral thesis

A doctoral thesis is a scholarly piece of work, normally of 70–100 000 words in length, which makes a significant contribution to the body of knowledge in a specialised field. It is expected that peers will evaluate the work as comparable to, or better than, work of a similar kind. It is difficult to describe the role and nature of the PhD exactly, because of substantial variations in their substance and character. In spite of this, Sheehan (1994) declares that, on the whole, consensus about quality in PhDs is possible and does exist. Phillips and Pugh (1994), and others such as Cowen (1997), recount some of the history and development of the PhD which we are unable to discuss here but may be of interest in relation to understanding these issues.

Most academics agree that, first and foremost, the PhD should make a distinct contribution to knowledge. For this, it is necessary for the candidate to demonstrate, either in the text or in the viva that they are fully aware of the existing state of knowledge. Readers of the study should recognise that the researcher has examined and presented alternative ideas and does not let personal prejudice and preferences interfere in the argument. Coherent and convincing arguments about the research problem and avoidance of irrelevant details and areas add to the quality of a thesis.

The PhD thesis, once examined and passed, is immediately placed in the public domain. It does not have to be a *magnum opus* (Lawton, 1997), but must be of publishable quality. The concept of 'publishability' has its root in nineteenth-century Germany where publication was required from doctoral candidates (Simpson, 1983). Indeed in many universities a PhD can still be awarded to staff on the basis of refereed published articles in reputable academic and professional journals (see p. 12).

Quality indicators for MPhil and PhD theses

The guidelines of the Higher Education Quality Council (HEQC, 1996) contain some of the major criteria on which research degrees are awarded. Students must demonstrate their competence through the production of a high-level, scholarly piece of research which advances the discipline within a particular time span. In health and social care disciplines, there may also be demands on students to advance professional practice. The indicators of quality comprise the following:

- A significant contribution to knowledge in the chosen field (PhD)
- Originality and creativity
- Independent work
- Critical and analytical thought
- Coherence and synthesis

The first indicator, a significant contribution to knowledge, is an essential component of the PhD but does not necessarily apply to the MPhil. The contribution refers to theoretical or methodological developments and/or new facts. It is often closely related to the concept of originality and creativity.

Originality is a difficult concept, often misunderstood and full of ambiguities when applied to PhD research. Locke *et al.* (1993) claim that much confusion exists in this area because academics as well as professionals interpret the term *original* research as that which has never occurred before and which is the first ground-breaking study in the field. Although this type of research can, of course, lay claim to originality according to this definition, most PhD studies do not achieve it.

Apart from the notion of originality mentioned above as 'first', 'completely new' (that which has not existed before), the concept can be broadened according to Phillips and Pugh (1994) and Cryer (1996) to mean:

- The use or development of new research instruments or techniques.
- Carrying out different types of sampling from those in previous research.
- Employing old instruments or techniques in a new area of study or a new setting.
- Using approaches different from those employed in previously completed studies.
- Bringing new theoretical perspectives to a field of study.

Creativity refers to the ability of the researcher to adopt a different or unusual stance. While this may be highly regarded if successful, some supervisors may see this as a high-risk strategy and encourage their students to adopt a safer, tried and tested approach which will assure a successful outcome.

MPhil and PhD research must show good evidence of independent work. One of the most difficult tasks of students is to carry out work which is seen to be independent from that of supervisors or other members of a research team. Some students experience difficulty in becoming independent of their supervisors whose initial guidance had helped them on their way. There will be a stage when students develop their own work in their own way and make critical judgements independent of supervisors, though still being influenced by the thinking and interaction with the supervisory team.

The nature of any thesis, but particularly a PhD thesis, demands a high level of conceptual, logical and theoretical thought, made explicit in the completed work. It is relatively common for students working in health and social care to focus great attention on the implications and applications of their study while neglecting the theoretical framework. The latter is essential for work at this level.

Coherence, integration and synthesis of all of the material is a fundamental requirement of MPhil and PhD theses. The aims, objectives,
rationale, research methods, findings and conclusions should relate to
each other in a logical progression or in a series of logical stages.
Reading completed theses is a useful way of becoming acquainted with
the nature of MPhil and PhD research. You will find out quickly that
very different styles of writing, conceptualisation and presentation exist
and that no thesis is entirely free of errors. Of course, someone else's
thesis can never be a 'template' for one's own (Fitzpatrick *et al.*, 1998).

The PhD award based on publications

Most PhDs are awarded to those proceeding through the traditional
route of registration and supervision. However, in many UK universities, a mechanism exists for gaining a doctorate by submitting a
body of published work. If you are interested in taking this route, you
must find out whether the university offers this type of PhD. In general,
you will have to be a member of staff, for example tutor, lecturer or
lecturer practitioner.

As a member of university staff who is also a health or social care
professional, this may be a good way of staying in touch with your
profession. It enables you to undertake research in your practice area and
publish regularly, as the work progresses, in peer-reviewed professional
and academic journals. The UK Council for Graduate Education (1996)
maintains that the PhD by publications is particularly useful for those
studying part-time and who have come into higher education at a mid-
stage in their careers. It specifically mentions, among others, individuals
in practice-based disciplines such as nursing and other professions allied
to medicine as well as social work.

The major differences between a PhD by the conventional route and
by published work include the following:

- The traditional PhD requires a thesis while the PhD by published
  work requires a series of publications.
- The traditional PhD is generally longer in terms of word count.
- Delays in acceptance and publication usually offset any potential
  time advantage to the publications route.
- The PhD by publications can be carried out without a supervisor,
  although most institutions allocate an adviser or mentor to the
  candidate.

- The training process for the PhD by publications is less formal in general.

An important advantage of following the publications route is that the production of tangible outputs in the form of published work enhances the individual's reputation and career prospects from an early stage of the research. The main disadvantage is that individuals rarely complete the volume of work necessary to submit for a PhD (often for the same reason!).

A number of factors are common to both types of PhD in most institutions:

- The research makes a contribution to knowledge.
- The postgraduate has been trained in the approved methodology.
- The candidate has in-depth knowledge of his or her area of research.
- The work should show that the research forms a coherent body of work.
- They are equally demanding and of comparable standard, coherence and quality.
- They are assessed by examination including a viva.
- All types of PhD research require demonstration of an independent contribution by the candidate.

The major common factor is the quality of the research, and this is why potential candidates are advised to seek academic advice at an early stage. The PhD by publications is open to public scrutiny through publication in high-quality journals which are refereed by academic peers, or in books which have been critically appraised by experts in the field. Candidates will obtain guidance on this from the regulations of the university and academic advisers. The candidates must normally submit a written rationale with their list of publications to the relevant research degrees committee in order to gain approval to submit for examination. In preparation for the examination itself, most institutions of higher education demand a summary or abstract, introductory chapter and supportive analysis with off-prints of photocopies of all publications so that the award can be considered. The examination and viva procedures are then similar to those for a conventional PhD (see Chapter 11). Apart from the assessment of the quality of the work, the methodology will be scrutinised in more detail because many publications only summarise and do not detail the type of approach as carefully and at such length as does a PhD thesis. The research committee will usually carry out the following:

- An evaluation of the coherence of the body of work.
- An assessment of the location of the work within the time frame and type of journal.
- An evaluation of the independent contribution of the candidate, if the publications have been written jointly with others.

The number of publications is not formally set by most institutions, though around ten articles of about 5000 words is the norm. The university may impose a time limit on the duration of the study and potential candidates are encouraged to check this at an early stage. The report prepared by Professor Keith Wilson published by the UK Council for Graduate Education (1996) provides further detail.

Taught and professional doctorates

Most, if not all, universities and their departments provide a programme of research training for their MPhil/PhD students. Some, however, offer a more lengthy programme of study for doctoral students. This programme often includes subject knowledge as well as issues of methodology. It is sometimes referred to as a *taught PhD*, although this is something of a misnomer as students do still have to produce an independent thesis. However, it differs from a conventional PhD through its substantial taught components and additional written assessments on such aspects as theory, methodology and data analysis.

Doctorates in business administration or education commonly contain such taught elements. Health and social care professionals working in management positions sometimes register for a Doctor of Business Administration (DBA) programme, while those interested in teaching and learning may register for a Doctor of Education (DEd). Some universities provide professional or practice-based doctorates for students who transfer from a taught Masters programme. The University of Ulster, for instance, has introduced a Doctor of Medical Science (DMedSci) which follows a vocational/professional route. Candidates submit projects of direct and practical relevance to their profession and also complete a thesis which contributes to knowledge in their field. At least three years of professional practice are mandatory before students can register for this type of doctorate. Most clinical psychology departments now offer courses for a Doctorate in Clinical Psychology (DClinPsychol) which are very competitive and exacting. These generally involve research training as well as professional clinical practice under supervision. Examination includes coursework assessments, a doctoral thesis based on original work, as well as a viva with both internal and external examiners.

With the growth of the new, more vocationally oriented universities, it is likely that more institutions will consider the development of professional or taught doctorates. It is necessary to think very carefully about the programme you wish to pursue and compare the options. While interim assessments might seem unnecessarily onerous and the final qualification sounds somewhat different from a PhD, those coming from a practitioner background may find the additional research training of substantial value.

References

Cowen, R. (1997) Comparative perspectives on the British PhD. In *Working for a Doctorate: a Guide for the Humanities and Social Sciences* (eds N. Graves & V. Varma), pp. 184–199. Routledge, London.

Cryer, P. (1996) *The Research Student's Guide to Success*. Open University Press, Buckingham.

Fitzpatrick, J., Secrist, J. & Wright D.J. (1998) *Secrets for a Successful Dissertation*. Sage, Thousand Oaks, CA.

HEQC (1996) *Guidelines on the Quality Assurance of Research Degrees*. Higher Education Quality Council, London.

Lawton, D. (1997) How to proceed in postgraduate study. In *Working for a Doctorate: a Guide for the Humanities and Social Sciences*. (eds N. Graves & V. Varma), pp. 1–17. Routledge, London.

Locke, L.F., Spirduso, W.W. & Silverman, S.J. (1993) *Proposals That Work: a Guide for Planning Dissertations and Grant Proposals*, 3rd edn. Sage, Newbury Park, CA.

McKenzie, G., Powell, J. & Usher, R. (1997) *Understanding Social Research: Perspectives on Methodology and Practice*. Falmer Press, London.

Phillips, E.M. & Pugh, D.S. (1994) *How to Get a PhD: a Handbook for Students and their Supervisors*, 2nd edn. Open University Press, Buckingham.

Sheehan, P. (1994) From thesis writing to research application. In *Quality in Postgraduate Education* (eds O. Zuber-Skerritt & Y. Ryan), pp. 14–23. Kogan Page, London.

Simpson, R. (1983) *How the PhD Came to Britain*. Society for Research in Higher Education, Guildford.

UK Council for Graduate Education (1996) *The Award of the Degree of PhD on the Basis of Published Work in the UK*. UKCGE, Warwick.

Further reading

Advisory Board for the Research Councils (1993) *The Nature of the PhD: a Discussion Document*. Office of Science and Technology, London.

Bargar, R.R. & Duncan, J.K. (1982) Cultivating creative endeavour in doctoral research. *Journal of Higher Education*, 53(1), 1–31.

The following are not books on research methods but are about debates in the philosophy of science.

Blaikie, N. (1993) *Approaches to Social Enquiry*. Polity Press, Cambridge.

Hughes, G. (1990) *The Philosophy of Social Science Research*, 2nd edn. Longman, London.

Layder, D. (1993) *New Strategies in Social Research: an Introduction and Guide*. Polity Press, Cambridge.

Thompson, N. (1995) *Theory and Practice in Health and Social Welfare*. Open University Press, Buckingham (in particular Chapter 3, Science and research).

Chapter 2

Preparing for Enrolment

Educational prerequisites

Many institutions require that candidates for an MPhil/PhD must hold a 'good' first degree (a 1st or 2 : 1) or a Masters qualification (preferably both) from a recognised awarding body. A first degree usually provides a more broad-based educational foundation, while a Masters qualification demonstrates mastery of a relevant discipline or topic area. Both include the development of critical and analytical thought. Exceptions are sometimes made in unusual circumstances for people with diplomas in research or those who have extensive research experience. In every case, you must demonstrate that you have the necessary knowledge base, including analytical and critical skills, as well as the ability and determination to conduct research at this level and develop and write a thesis.

Most, though not all, of those carrying out research in health or social care hold professional qualifications – it is usually this which has stimulated their interest in a particular topic. But a professional qualification alone is insufficient preparation for study at this level. If you wish to proceed to a PhD you should ensure that you are able to demonstrate the following:

- Mastery of at least some of the key theories or debates of relevance to the topic under study.
- Skills in critically analysing and summarising a broad research-based literature.
- Academic writing and reporting skills.
- Basic knowledge of research methods and their applications, and the philosophy of science (at least to level 3).
- Overwhelming curiosity, and enthusiasm for the topic and the process of inquiry.

Students with a professional qualification, even if they have some research experience, often lack the academic background that will

17

enable them to analyse issues critically from different perspectives and consider the full range of research possibilities available. Such individuals may benefit either from extending their educational preparation, for example through a taught Masters programme which includes a research-based dissertation, or from enrolling on a taught doctoral programme. You should consider these issues carefully with academic advisers before registering for a research degree.

Sound knowledge of at least one relevant social science (e.g. psychology, sociology, anthropology) is very useful for research into any aspect of health or social care, depending on the topic in question. An educational background in one of these is likely to stimulate students to question the nature of truth and authenticity and encourage them to look outside the health or social care literature for different ideas, theoretical perspectives, research literature and methodologies. Even professionals using traditional experimental designs need to take full account of human understanding and social context in assessing the implications of their research.

Students with a first degree in the social sciences often compete with those from professional backgrounds for full-time studentships to study issues related to health and social care. These students usually have the advantage of being younger and more willing to survive on a small research grant. On the other hand, those from relevant professional backgrounds are advantaged by their 'insider' knowledge about health and social care systems, how they operate, who the gatekeepers are, the nature of the culture, the terminology or jargon used, service priorities and ethical procedures. They often have good communication skills, confidence in dealing with people in a variety of contexts, are motivated to persevere in the face of difficulties, and have the ability to work autonomously. For these reasons, those with professional or academic backgrounds in health and social care are usually welcome applicants for research degrees.

Institutions accepting students for a higher degree usually try to ensure that these are properly equipped with the necessary knowledge and skills before they start, but also offer a suitable programme of training and seminars to build up their knowledge base and confidence before and during the period of study. In our experience, all institutions are very careful in their selection of full-time students, not least because the research funding councils have imposed strict guidelines on completion rates and times, which they monitor carefully. However, some supervisors are less careful about the selection of part-time students. If you are willing to pay the fees, institutions may be happy to enrol you with few questions asked. Even experienced professionals feel flattered if a senior academic offers them the opportunity to study for a higher degree. But you are advised to proceed cautiously. Completion rates for part-time students are much lower, and resubmission and failure rates higher, than those for full-time students, particularly among those who are ill prepared educationally.

A cautionary tale – this is based on a genuine case, though many details have been changed to preclude the possibility of recognition.

Don was a nurse with a Diploma in Professional Studies. He had already built up a national reputation in his clinical speciality when a well-known senior academic encouraged him to register part-time for a PhD in order to demonstrate the importance of a particular aspect of his work. His eventual submission for the PhD failed for a number of reasons. The thesis demonstrated a lack of fairly basic skills in academic writing, a lack of understanding of a sufficiently broad theoretical literature, and a lack of evidence of high-level skills in critical reasoning and evaluation. In other words, the thesis was poorly expressed, superficial and biased. Don had enrolled at a centre of excellence a considerable travelling distance from home and, although he had attended the research training days offered, had not been able to engage fully in the research culture of the department. There were fundamental flaws in the research design which had not been recognised early on and were later irredeemable. Although the supervisor knew the thesis to be weak, she was sympathetic to the length of time it had taken to produce (seven years), the student's current work pressures and lack of motivation caused by the substantial amendments already made. She finally agreed to submission in the belief that redemption would be possible. Outright failure had a devastating impact on them both in terms of personal recrimination and professional status. In this case, there were found to be no reasonable grounds for appeal, though the university subsequently changed its admission policy to exclude those without a first or higher degree.

It often seems unnecessarily onerous for experienced health or social care professionals to have to take a further course of study when what they really want to do is to solve important practice-based problems. There is usually an academic somewhere who is willing to give them the opportunity to register for a higher degree (and take their fees and their ideas). Seeking to undertake a research degree without traditional educational preparation is a high-risk strategy which can sometimes pay off (see the second example in the Epilogue) but may lead to heartache and failure. You should think very carefully if it is really worthwhile taking short cuts.

Locating the topic

When studying for an MPhil, but more particularly a PhD in health or social care, you need to decide at an early stage where to locate yourself in terms of philosophical perspective, academic tradition, professional application and academic department. Further consideration is given to these issues in Chapter 3. However, many of these issues are closely interrelated and each can have a profound influence on the choice of supervisor, the nature of the PhD, external examiner and future career trajectory.

In order to illustrate more fully the implications of these issues, we have used an example of the study of the cerebral vascular accident (CVA or stroke). Professionals working in the sphere of health or social care may choose to locate their study of CVA in one or any combination of the following perspectives. Examples of some of the relevant disciplines are given in parentheses merely to illustrate the potential range of choice facing the student. They are not, of course, intended to be definitive.

Incidence and aetiology of stroke (public health medicine, epidemiology, medical statistics)

Brain function (neuroscience, cognitive science, radiography, computing, biological science)

Genetics (biological/clinical science, social psychology, moral philosophy)

Rehabilitation (occupational therapy, physiotherapy, speech therapy, sports science, rehabilitation studies, biotechnology, communication studies, education studies, disability studies)

Nutritional state (nutritional science, dietetics, health science, nursing studies, social psychology)

Communication (social psychology, speech therapy, computer science and technology)

Social impact (sociology, social work studies, disability studies, gerontology)

Psychological impact (psychophysiology, cognitive science, health psychology, clinical psychology, counselling, linguistics)
Care/carer issues (social work studies, gerontological nursing, mental health nursing, community studies, health psychology)
Policy (health policy studies, social studies, social policy, politics)
Death and bereavement (nursing studies, social work studies, counselling, sociology, psychology)

A PhD in the social sciences is likely to be very different from one based in the biological, medical or health sciences. Students who wish to integrate different aspects may experience particular difficulties choosing an appropriate university department and supervisory team.

In making a decision, you are likely to be guided by the following:

- The nature of your existing degrees
- Your knowledge of particular universities, departments and supervisors
- Discussion with and advice from 'experts' in the field
- Your philosophical stance (e.g. positivist, feminist, post-modern)
- The type of approach and methodology you wish to use
- Special resources required
- Access and ethical issues
- Qualifications desired
- Ultimate career choice

A university department, in deciding to accept you, would usually take account of:

- The nature of your existing degrees
- Availability of suitable supervisory support
- Availability of suitable resources to support the research
- The contribution of your research to the departmental Research Assessment Exercise (RAE) aspirations
- The willingness of the institution/department/supervisor to entertain cross-disciplinary collaboration
- Evidence of your motivation and ability to work effectively and autonomously

You should be aware that you do not have to be a social worker to register for a postgraduate research degree in a social work studies department, nor a nurse to register in a nursing department.

Example

Jill, a midwife, wished to study family experiences of having a baby and was encouraged to register in a department of social work studies which specialised in family studies using the type of methodologies in which she was interested. The department was able to provide help in obtaining funds to support her part-time fees and she was delighted to find herself in a research community rich in new ideas about social aspects of family life.

You need to be aware that decisions you make about the location of your study can influence the nature of your final qualifications and your career choice. For example, Jan Walker was delighted to find out after she had obtained her PhD that she was eligible to register with the British Psychological Society (BPS) as a chartered psychologist and practising health psychologist. This was because she had a first degree in psychology which had BPS recognition, her PhD had been supervised and, more importantly, examined by a psychologist, and she was able to provide evidence of sufficient practical experience of applied health psychology before, during and after her PhD. Chartered practitioner status not only gave her an additional professional qualification but direct access to additional career opportunities.

Choosing a university and department

Decisions are likely to be influenced by a number of factors. Full-time students might be affected by the availability of funded studentships, while part-time students are more likely to be influenced by location. Both will require expert supervision. Departments such as psychology often have a history of success in attracting full-time funded studentships and providing expert supervision. However, some are increasingly reluctant to enrol students from other disciplines or areas of study. This is largely because of the current pressures on university staff to publish in journals which carry high kudos in their specific subject area for the Research Assessment Exercise. In addition, students without a first degree in the discipline of the department in which they register can find themselves out of their depth in terms of theoretical knowledge and inadequate in relation to their new peers.

Example

Jackie, a former midwife with a degree in sociology and a Masters in midwifery was very interested in carrying out PhD research with a large element of psychology which she wanted to develop. She decided to enrol in the psychology department of a traditional university. The department demanded that Jackie undertake a Masters degree in psychology first. Jackie, in her mid-40s, was loathe to spend two more years on another Masters degree, revised her ideas and enrolled in the midwifery department of a new university where she was supervised by a midwifery lecturer and a psychologist from the psychology department in the same faculty.

If you have freedom of choice, because you will be paying your own fees, you should weigh up the following issues. These are far from clear-cut:

- *Location.* There are clear advantages to having convenient access to supervisor, research training programme, library and computing facilities. Access to academics is often difficult enough even at close quarters and can get more trying as the study progresses.

- *Prestige.* There are advantages to gaining a higher degree from a well-established and recognised institution with well-known academics. However, they do not always have the time or inclination to devote to the needs of part-time or mature students.

- *Support systems.* Well-established institutions usually offer a wider network of research contacts, seminars given by international experts, and well-established support systems (research training, information technology (IT), statistical help, etc.). On the other hand, smaller and less well-known institutions may try to compensate by generous nurturing of their research students.

- *Experienced supervision.* Many small colleges and new universities find it difficult to provide experienced supervision in the fields of health and social care. On the other hand, most try to compensate by ensuring that inexperienced supervisors have adequate support, from outside if necessary, and attend training courses in supervision.

- *Discipline*. Locating oneself outside one's own discipline may appear academically advantageous, but can lead to feelings of academic and social isolation.

- *Size*.   Larger institutions and departments provide a bigger critical mass of researchers and research students, offering a richer research community. Smaller institutions and departments may try to compensate for the lack of this by offering good study facilities and more individual attention from supervisors.

Students wishing to make use of highly specialised equipment or expertise will naturally be more limited in scope in their choice of academic department. It is important to ensure that the facilities likely to be needed are available at the time of application and do not rely on funding applications which may not succeed, or on collaboration with other organisations or institutions for which explicit permission has not been given. Written undertakings *must* be obtained before any commitment can be assumed.

Evaluating the research environment

It is important to consider the research culture in the relevant department or faculty. Sometimes students complain that they work in a vacuum in isolation from others. Therefore, it is sensible to examine the research strategy or policies of the institution or department and the way research-active staff members work together and with their students. Newbury (1996) expressed the view of many researchers that 'Students benefit from being part of a community of research students' (p. 19). If this does not happen, students do not learn from the experience of peers nor have they contact with others outside their own discipline and area of study. This is, of course, much more difficult for part-time than for full-time students. Both need to be assured of the quality of research supervision they are likely to receive.

The following are considered to be minimum requirements for research supervision in most higher education institutions:

- The supervisory team should, between them, have supervised at least two PhDs (or MPhils if students are studying to MPhil) to completion.
- The director of studies or first supervisor should not be registered for a PhD.

- Other supervisors with relevant experience and expertise may be registered for their own PhD, but there should be no possible conflict of interest.
- None of the supervisors should be supervising more than five full-time equivalent (FTE) research students.
- Academic members of the supervisory team should be actively engaged in their own programme of research and publication (ask to see a curriculum vitae or publication record).
- The supervisory team should ideally include at least one person (who may act as an adviser) with a strong background in health or social care who understands the particular demands imposed within the field of application.
- The director of studies should demonstrate commitment to the student through the regular allocation of time. The students should check if they are planning to spend time abroad and what will happen if or when they take sabbatical leave.
- Full-time students should be provided with a desk and locker in an office (usually shared), the use of a computer with appropriate software, internet and e-mail connections.
- Part-time students should be given access to computing facilities with internet access.
- The library should provide a basic range of books and journals on the topic area and research methods, appropriate literature search facilities, and interlibrary loan facilities for specialised material.
- There should be adequate statistical support and data analysis software available, as necessary, for the research.
- There should be an induction, research training and seminar programme for students to attend. Part-time students should ensure that they will be able to attend most or some of these.
- Full-time students may be requested to act as a teaching assistant or demonstrator. This should not involve management responsibilities or extensive preparation and should not normally exceed six hours per week. (Some institutions now provide some basic training in teaching and learning strategies to facilitate this.)

It is always a good idea to ask to speak informally with other research students to find out about their experiences before making a decision. The following questions are relevant:

- Does the supervisor provide adequate attention, encouragement and support?

- Are the available facilities adequate to support their research?
- Are research students able to communicate with each other and present their ideas in a common forum?
- Does a good working climate and atmosphere of enthusiasm permeate the department?
- Do the rest of the staff members value and appreciate research?

Understanding the context of higher education

The context of higher education is quite different from that of service-based organisations. It is helpful if you have some basic knowledge of this before you start so that you understand some of the rules and constraints you may have to face.

Research funding in higher education

University departments have a limited range of sources of income for research. These include:

(1) The Higher Education Funding Council for England (HEFCE) – Research funding from this source is capped to ensure that universities do not divert money intended for teaching into research (this applies also to the Scottish Higher Education Funding Council, the Higher Education Funding Council for Wales and the Department of Education Northern Ireland).
(2) HEFCE funding from the Research Assessment Exercise (see below).
(3) External research project funding from research councils, the National Health Service Executive (NHSE) and charitable bodies. Applications are submitted from individual researchers or research groups.
(4) Full-time studentships and part-time bursaries funded by research councils and the NHSE and awarded on the basis of competitive tender to university departments.
(5) Part-time student fees.

It is important to note that research is a costly business, not least in terms of researcher time. Few university departments make a profit from it, but most wish to use it to raise their profile in order to attract high-calibre staff and students. Departments with service education contracts may be in a better financial position to subsidise their research activities and enable staff to support research students with a higher standard of accommodation and equipment (including computers), while well-established universities usually offer a higher level of technical (including statistical) support.

The Research Assessment Exercise

The impact of the RAE on university departments cannot be overstated. The RAE was conducted in 1992 and 1996 and will be repeated in 2001. It involves the setting up of panels of experts in 69 discrete subject areas (or units of assessment). In addition to traditional 'pure' subject areas, a number of clinically based subjects of relevance to medicine, nursing (including midwifery and health visiting), 'other studies and professions allied to medicine', social work and social policy are included. Each university department must decide if it wishes its research to be assessed and, if so, which panel is most appropriate. Details of research-based publications by staff, together with research funding received and students supervised and completed must be submitted. The panel awards a score from 1 (little research activity of any national significance) to 5* (all research activity is of international importance). This score is then multiplied by the number of staff entered and the extent of research activities to determine the funding allocated for future research from the HEFCE. Thus the potential rating must be traded off against potential funding income. A department which obtains a high score is viewed favourably by the funding authorities, including the NHSE, so that success breeds success.

Departments specialising in health and social care have tended to attract low RAE ratings, largely because they are relatively new to research and have yet to build up a critical mass of experienced researchers. Without a strong research culture, the research may or may not be of the highest quality. Many nursing departments, for instance, chose not to enter into the 1996 RAE, or scored only 1. Students may wish to consider this when applying to register for a higher degree at a lesser-known institution. However, there is much game-playing within this system which can lead to winners and losers who, in reality, appear little different to each other. For example, experienced and well-established institutions with an eye firmly on the future tended to enter only a few select members of staff who were likely to attract a high rating. Others chose to maximise future funding by using the multiplier and traded large numbers of staff against a lower rating.

The Harris Report

The Harris Report (1996) recommended minimum standards for research in higher education, including the nature of the research environment. They include:

- A critical mass of active research staff working in the field of study.
- An RAE rating indicative of high-quality research.
- A critical mass of research students working in the field of study.
- A compulsory research training programme for all postgraduate research students.
- A programme of seminars involving at least some external speakers during the year.

Some universities have been more rigid in their interpretation and implementation of Harris than others. Several traditional universities have stipulated that students may be supervised only where there is a critical mass of at least ten research-active staff and an RAE grading of 4. Many new universities are not yet able to meet standards relating to RAE ratings and critical mass. Most departments in the field of health and social care fall below these requirements, though many succeed, nevertheless, in producing good results for their students. You need to judge for yourself what is on offer but may wish to bear these recommendations in mind when judging the academic strength of a department.

Opportunities for funding

You may wish to apply for funding to study full-time for the research degree or help with payment of fees or research expenses. The best ways to find out about potential funding sources are (not necessarily in this order):

(1) *Health and social care organisations*
    (a) Mail shots to academic departments
    (b) Internet websites

(2) *Professional bodies*
    (a) Advertisements in professional journals
    (b) Professional mailing to individuals
    (c) Mail shots to academic departments
    (d) Internet websites

(3) *Research councils*
  (a) Studentships are normally advertised by academic departments

(4) *Large charities*
  (a) Advertisements in *Education Guardian, Times Higher Education*
  (b) Supplement (*Times Higher Education Supplement*), professional journals
  (c) Mailing to academic institutions, departments and individuals
  (d) Digests – available in libraries
  (e) Internet websites

(5) *Small charities*
  (a) Personal knowledge and contact (of student and/or supervisor)
  (b) Digests – available from libraries

A guide to grant applications has been published by BMJ Books (Crombie & du V Florey, 1998). This book gives an overview of the process of application, guidelines for writing an application and a number of contact addresses for health and medical research in particular, but also for social research.

If you apply to the **NHSE** for funding, you should be aware that the NHS has developed a national strategy for research and development. This was in recognition that the large amount of NHS money spent each year on research had yielded little in the way of innovations in practice and improvements in patient care. Some key points of interest to emerge from this strategy were:

(1) An emphasis on multidisciplinary research. This means that no money is set aside for individual groups of practitioners such as nurses or professions allied to medicine (PAMS).
(2) Funding priorities are determined at national and local levels. Information, including addresses, can be found on the internet.
(3) Direct medical research funding is allocated on the basis of the quality of the research undertaken (rather than as of right).
(4) Funding is available for individual projects, on a competitive basis, from NHSE Research and Development (R&D) directorate. Details are available from regional offices by telephone, e-mail or website.

To find out about regional NHS funding you can search on the website: the search term is *NHS Executive R&D*; then click on *NHSE R&D Directorates*; then select the one to gain access to the home page.

Some professional bodies and organisations, such as the Central Council for Education and Training in Social Work (**CCETSW**) help to fund research through the payment of course fees or expenses, though this may be restricted to those registered in approved departments. Some organisations, such as training hospitals, have educational trusts which provide small one-off grants; for example, to assist with course fees, purchasing specialist books, or conference attendance.

In the UK, a number of research councils fund quality projects in the relevant areas. All councils have similar conditions of eligibility for students, and these include: graduates with first or upper-second class degrees from a UK higher education institution; the institution must be approved and recognised by the particular council. Other conditions of eligibility exist and applications are assessed on merit.

The **Medical Research Council** (MRC) funds all forms of biomedical research, but it is very difficult for research students, particularly those in the new universities, to gain funding from this source.

The **Economic and Social Research Council** (ESRC) provides postgraduate studentships in the social sciences. This includes innovative research of relevance to health and social care. To gain such studentships, PhD students must attend a university department whose research environment and education and training has been approved by the ESRC. ESRC materials, with details on studentship awards and applications are available in the 'Guidance Notes for Applicants' issued annually to the registry or central administration offices of higher education institutions. They include information about ESRC's support for full-time and part-time students and how they can apply. These materials along with lists of ESRC-recognised outlets, courses and programmes are signposted on the Internet at: http://www.esrc.ac.uk/ptd/ptd.html.

The ESRC has some general criteria for institutions which concern in the main the adequacy of formal training in research methodologies, the adequacy of supervision arrangements and the importance of an active research environment, as well as an adequate critical mass of students who can benefit by interaction with peers.

Other councils provide similar funding opportunities.

The **Biotechnology and Biological Science Research Council** (BBSRC) funds projects in the fields of relevance to its title.

It is less likely that health and social care professionals will gain grants from the other councils although there may be possibilities depending on the research topic.

Many other grant-giving bodies exist, some of which also fund research training. For example, the **Nuffield Foundation** funds small self-contained projects with relevance to practice and policy including health and social care. The **Joseph Rowntree Foundation** funds research on housing, social care, social policy and disability. The **Kings Fund**, the **Wellcome Trust**, the **Nuffield Provincial Hospitals Trust** and the **Association of Medical Charities**, to name but a few, are some of the non-government agencies which fund health research. Most of these publish an annual report to provide information and guidance for those wishing to apply for grants. The Association of Medical Charities publishes an annual handbook listing grant-giving agencies, with particular reference to areas where there is overlap between health and social care (for instance, the Alzheimer Disease Society, the Mental Health Foundation, the Muscular Dystrophy Group). Many charities, housing trusts and foundations give small grants to research students if these can make a good case that their research is necessary. Those undertaking community-based action research may consider applying for European funding. Expert help is normally necessary for this as competition is strong and the process is quite lengthy.

You will find addresses and compendia in the library of your university. If you enrol in a department which specialises in health, community or social care, the addresses will probably be available within the department or faculty. The Internet is an increasingly important source of research funding opportunities including details of funding criteria, guidelines for applicants, submission deadlines, and applications. Researchers can access these via search engines, using search commands which target general topic areas or, more effectively, specific organisations (such as the NHSE or CCETSW).

Applications for full-time funding should be made prior to registration for a research degree. Some agencies will not consider applications from students who have already registered (see p. 32), even though they must demonstrate that they have a supervisor/department/university willing to accept them.

Another way of being funded is by accepting a research assistant post. Research assistants are salaried members of university staff who have research and some teaching duties (the latter should be very limited). Your own research may be a development or part of the research work you are carrying out for the university. However, research funding for the post rarely lasts longer than three years, and your own study will suffer from conflicting demands, researching and teaching for the university and progressing in your own PhD work.

Enrolment and registration

You should note that registration for a higher degree is quite separate from enrolment. Enrolment is the point at which the university starts charging fees and allows you full access to its facilities including supervision, library and information technology. Registration refers to the date at which the university accepts you as a registered candidate for MPhil/PhD, having demonstrated that you fulfil all of the requirements necessary for study at this level, including the presentation of a suitable plan of investigation. Since most universities are prepared to backdate registration, the date of registration may coincide with the date of enrolment, particularly for full-time students. However, if time has been spent since enrolment in preparation, applying for research funds, negotiating access or ethical approval, the date of enrolment may precede the date of registration by some months. This preparation time should be regarded as time well spent, since any time limit imposed by the university on completion of the MPhil or PhD relates to the period of registration and not enrolment. Although most universities stipulate a minimum time to completion, few actually delay the submission of a finished thesis where there is sound evidence of independent work.

References

Crombie I.K. & du V Florey, C. (1998) *A Pocket Guide to Grant Applications.* BMJ Publishing, London.

Harris, M. (1996) *Review of Postgraduate Education.* The Higher Education Council for England, Bristol (The Harris Report).

Newbury, D. (1996) *Doing a Postgraduate Degree: a Research Guide.* Birmingham Institute of Art and Design, Birmingham

Further reading

Bourner, T. & Race, P. (1990) *How to Win as a Part-Time Student.* Kogan Page, London.

National Postgraduate Committee (1995a) *Guidelines for Code of Practice for Postgraduate Research*. Brandon House, Troon.

National Postgraduate Committee (1995b) *The Postgraduate Book*, 2nd edn. Brandon House, Troon.

Chapter 3

Research Supervision

The choice of supervisors

Choosing a supervisor is probably the most important decision you will have to make, assuming that you have a choice. The research supervisor is the person with particular expertise in the relevant area of study or methodology, who oversees the general progress of MPhil or PhD research. He or she not only advises on the research itself, both in the area of study and methodology, but also guides and supports you through the maze of regulations and rules of your university. The experience and expertise of the supervisor can influence the eventual quality of the thesis and its success or failure. However, it is the quality of the relationship that you establish with your supervisors which is most likely to determine whether or not you actually complete and submit the thesis. A good relationship with the supervisors will see you through most difficulties. A poor relationship is a recipe for disaster and can, from our observations, end in demoralisation and depression, as well as failure to complete.

There may be no choice of supervisor. For example, if you apply for an established research studentship, the supervisor and research topic will already be determined. It is very flattering to be offered such a studentship, but you should think carefully about whether you will be able to live (metaphorically) with the topic and the supervisor for a minimum of three years full-time, or between four and seven years part-time.

If you wish to research a topic of your choice and apply to become a part-time student, or want help in applying for a funded studentship (such as those granted by the NHS), there are a number of ways of setting about this. If you have recently completed a first or Masters degree, you may already have a good relationship with an academic who is willing to support you, or help you to locate a suitable supervisor. Alternatively, you may know, by reputation or personal contact, of an academic you can approach for such assistance. If you are not familiar with suitable academic institutions or departments, such information can be found in the local library or on the Internet. You may then write to the academic registrar or to the head of department. In these circumstances, the head of department, senior researcher, postgraduate tutor or research committee will probably allocate you to an academic who is deemed to have the necessary expertise. You may or may not find this supervisor suitable.

Example

Jo, a nurse with experience of research and knowledge of a range of methodologies, applied at her local university to read for a PhD after completing a Master of Science programme. She had used quantitative measures in her MSc dissertation and intended to develop a phenomenological study of patient experiences and feelings about a chronic illness which seriously affects their lives. The university allocated a single supervisor who had some expertise in the area of chronic illness but not much knowledge of qualitative research. When she asked for an alternative supervisor with knowledge of this approach, the postgraduate tutor in the department reassured her that she would be able to use her chosen methodology, but that the university was not willing to change her supervisor. The student accepted this but found in the course of the first three months that the supervisor had no sympathy with her approach and advised her to use a different methodology. The student eventually changed universities to find a supervisor who had not only the expertise in the field of study but also the requisite knowledge of phenomenology. In the course of this process, the student lost three important months for her study.

If you are unsure about the supervisor you have been allocated you might negotiate for someone more suitable, or try another academic institution or department (don't forget that the Open University also offers PhD supervision), and see how they compare. Remember that as a potential research student with a good academic record you will enhance the research profile of any academic department and are there-fore a potentially valuable commodity. Make sure that your supervisor recognises your worth.

Sometimes students are allowed to choose their own supervisors from a list which includes their specific interests and methodological expertise. The freedom to choose can be useful for both student and supervisor since each needs to feel comfortable with the topic and the relationship. For supervisors, too, the selection process is important because of the close connections that will develop over time. Students require supervisors with whom they can work, who are seen as helpful and supportive, and who they respect as knowledgeable professionals.

We would strongly advise you to *interview* prospective supervisors before enrolling, to ascertain the following:

(1) Do the potential supervisors seem willing to listen to your ideas or do they appear too rigid or set in their ideas? Remember, it will eventually be your MPhil or PhD, not theirs.

(2) Do they appear to be on the same wavelength, or do they try to direct you towards a theoretical framework or methodological approach which feels quite wrong for your particular study?

(3) Is the supervisor enthusiastic about the research project? Enthusiasm can be very motivating.

(4) Is the supervisor interested in, or understanding of the importance of, the practice or professional applications of your work?

(5) How many students has the supervisor supervised to successful completion? A track record of success is an advantage, though too many may signal a production line approach.

(6) How many research students does the first supervisor have at the present time? Up to three or four others can be advantageous in terms of peer support. Any more may be a sign of overload, and the supervisor may lack time for individual attention.

(7) Find out how much time the supervisor intends to devote to your supervision. Some institutions have an agreed policy on this, while others do not. An average of an hour a week, at least, is a reasonable guide – this will include helping you to prepare the research proposal in the early stages, and reading and commenting on draft sections later on. Of course, supervision time will vary depending on the stage of the research.

(8) Find out if the supervisor is likely to take sabbatical leave during the course of your study, and, if so, what supervisory arrangements will be made for you. Some agree to continue supervising while others do not.

(9) Ask to speak to existing or former students to ascertain their supervisory experience and find out how long they are taking to complete (if some appear to be taking longer than expected, try to discover why).

(10)   Do you come away from these meetings with fresh ideas, feeling stimulated and motivated? If not, look around for someone else, if this is possible.

Single or joint supervision?

Some universities have the tradition of a single supervisor for a student, but most higher education institutions now have a small thesis advisory team for each doctoral candidate. Often the supervisory team consists of a director of studies, a second supervisor and/or an adviser who may be located outside the institution. The first supervisor has the main responsibility for the supervision of the study. The supervisory team must complement each other in terms of skills and knowledge.

There are a number of arguments for joint supervision:

(1)   For the student, continuity is ensured when one supervisor is absent, ill or leaves the university. In universities and colleges where members of staff move frequently, students will be safer with at least two supervisors.
(2)   The supervisors gain support from colleagues who can discuss the work of the student in terms of research methodology or topic area.
(3)   New supervisors go through an apprenticeship where they can obtain the guidance of experienced colleagues.

To avoid conflicting advice to students it is, of course, important that joint supervisors share ideas about supervision, have similar perspectives on the particular method and topic, and maintain contact with each other. It is advisable for the whole team to meet at least once a term or semester.

There is a need to match the style as well as the interests of supervisors and student. At the level of MPhil and PhD, it is expected that you work independently most of the time. Nevertheless, some supervisors expect you to submit work according to a mutually agreed timetable with clearly defined goals, while others adopt a more *laissez-faire* approach. Some students choose to work in a structured way, while others prefer to work at their own pace and see supervisors as an informal sounding board. It is useful to agree on these issues before starting the research.

Supervisors in the field of health and social care

For health and social care professionals who wish to obtain a higher degree in their own discipline, it is desirable, though not essential, that at least one member of the supervisory team has a similar professional background. But professionals with appropriate academic experience may be hard to find. Sociology, psychology and biology are academic disciplines which have a long tradition of study at doctoral level and a large number of academics with a research qualification. However, in disciplines such as nursing and the professions allied to medicine and social work, fewer PhDs have been obtained in the past, and the value of academic and theoretical work has been acknowledged only relatively recently. This means that there is likely to be a scarcity of experienced academic supervisors to suit your needs, leading to a difficult choice. On the one hand, you may be offered an inexperienced supervisor in a department which lacks a strong research culture and where there are few other research students. Universities can compensate for this, in collaboration with another institution, by selecting an external supervisor or adviser to provide the necessary supervisory experience and expertise. Most external supervisors receive only token payment and undertake this work primarily out of interest. On the other hand, you may elect to locate yourself in an academic discipline outside your professional discipline and recruit advisers from within your profession.

Example

Alison, a social worker, was offered an externally funded studentship in a well-established psychology department for research into elderly people with Alzheimer's disease, even though she did not have a first degree in psychology. As her ideas developed, she found that her interests in the management of cognitively impaired elderly people increasingly diverged from those of her supervisor, who was interested primarily in cognitive processing. The supervisor was under pressure to produce work related to pure (as opposed to applied) psychology since this was more likely to score high in the department's RAE ratings. Luckily, Alison was eventually successful in balancing her interests with those of her supervisor, but it was not easy.

The role of supervisors

Although supervision may differ according to circumstances – that is, the type of research and the topic, as well as the ability and experience of students – the principles remain similar for different students and types of research. Sharp and Howard (1996) claim that supervisors have some responsibility for the standard and completion of the research and for ensuring that students define and achieve aims and objectives. Supervisors and students have a common aim, that is to achieve a study of high standard which will be completed on time. The student and supervisor(s), respectively, should be committed to doing and supporting the research.

Supervisors have a number of responsibilities:

- Introduce their research students to the university, department and peers.
- Support and advise the student.
- Ensure that the student adheres to ethical principles.
- Offer criticism, where appropriate, in a constructive and encouraging manner.
- Ensure that students have adequate facilities and resources for their work.
- Ensure that students receive appropriate research training.
- Produce progress reports and be accountable to their departments.
- If there is an area of study in which they lack expertise, they are responsible for introducing students to other experts for advice.
- Encourage students to become part of the research student team.

Although it is not necessary that all members of the supervisory team have a PhD themselves, it is advisable that at least one has obtained this degree. It has been established that supervisors with doctoral experience have a higher level of involvement, a factor linked to success (Younman, 1992), although there may be exceptions.

The responsibilities of students

The ground rules are negotiated by supervisors and student at the very beginning of the relationship. Indeed, many institutions demand a formal contract between students and supervisors which sets out the terms of their professional relationship. Many relevant details can be found in the research student handbook (see Chapter 8), and it is a good idea to ask for a copy of this at an early stage.

The guidelines of the HEQC (1996) list a number of responsibilities for research students (to which others have been added). You are advised to:

- Negotiate your programme of study with your main supervisor and keep the supervisor regularly informed of all developments.
- Give written progress reports on the study to your supervisory team and the appropriate research committee, as required.
- Negotiate major changes and modifications of your study with the supervisors.
- Submit written sections or summaries of your work before regular supervisory meetings.
- Discuss academic problems related to the research with a view to their speedy resolution.
- Inform the supervisors of any personal or practical problems which might interfere with the smooth running of the research process.
- Attend agreed research training programmes.
- Observe ethical principles at all times.

The frequency of contact between you and the supervisor(s) depends on need and the stage of the research process. It should be negotiated at the beginning of the research and revised at intervals. Generally students need most help and support at the start and then again at the stage of writing up. Nevertheless, it is advisable to be in touch regularly throughout rather than at irregular and erratic intervals. Some people need to see the supervisor often, others enjoy working on their own though they, too, need feedback and constructive criticism. There should be a systematic and structured programme of work which forms the basis for the student–supervisor work relationship, but the instigation for this programme should come from you.

Phillips and Pugh (1994) list and discuss some of the expectations supervisors have of their students. The most important are the following:

- Supervisors expect students to consider their advice.
- Supervisors expect to be kept informed about student progress.
- Supervisors expect their students to start writing from an early stage.
- Supervisors expect a large measure of independence from students.

The responsibility for contacting supervisors rests largely with you. Telephone or e-mail contact can be useful, especially when you experience an academic or personal problem which affects the smooth process of the research and has to be resolved immediately.

The supervisor generally advises the student to come with questions and problems. Sharp and Howard (1996) advise that students inform the supervisor in advance of a meeting about the questions and problems they have. This means that both student and supervisor are prepared for the meeting, which saves precious time for all the participants. Supervisors are usually very involved and interested in the students' research topics and students have the right to expect this. Students and supervisors should keep written notes on the supervision meetings. This is useful as a basis for further appointments and makes meetings more systematic and methodical. You might find it useful to tape-record supervisory meetings, particularly during the final writing-up stage, though you should consult first with those involved in the meeting and ask for their permission. It is usual for the first supervisor to check the thesis when the final draft is finished to make sure of the level and coherence of the thesis, though he or she cannot be expected to correct spelling or referencing errors.

Students do not always want to begin writing before the start of the data collection; they believe that much of the research is 'in their head'. This is a fallacy, and it is useful for you to start writing early. The supervisor often asks for chapters on background, literature review and methodology, depending on the type of research, thus ensuring that you not only understand the process but also produce some ideas which generate fresh motivation and interest, even though sections of the writing might have to be changed at a later stage. This way you will be immersed in the study, you will have the opportunity to familiarise yourself with the details of the adopted methods. Some of the problems and pitfalls of the research then become obvious and can be resolved at an early stage.

Checklist for successful supervision

- Seek a first supervisor who is knowledgeable in your field and whose interests in the topic area and methodology matches yours.
- Confirm that the members of the supervisory team have enough time for your needs.

- Suggest the inclusion of a professional in your area of study as one of the members of your supervisory team.
- Try to get on with your supervisors.
- Negotiate and enter a contract with your supervisors.
- Be self-motivated and independent but do take advice and act on it.
- Fix meetings in advance and be scrupulous about timekeeping.
- Provide written work before and take notes during the meeting.
- Educate your supervisors.

(Problems with supervision will be discussed in Chapter 9.)

References

HEQC (1996) *Guidelines on the Quality Assurance of Research Degrees.* Higher Education Quality Council, London.

Phillips, E.M. & Pugh, D.S. (1994) *How to Get a PhD: a Handbook for Students and their Supervisors*, 2nd edn. Open University Press, Buckingham.

Sharp, J.A. & Howard, K. (1996) *The Management of a Student Research Project*, 2nd edn. Gower, Aldershot.

Youngman, M. (1992) Supervisors' and Students' Perceptions of Roles. Paper given at *Conference on Research Training in the Social Sciences*, St John's College, Cambridge, 11–12 September, 1992.

Further reading

Delamont, S., Atkinson, P. & Parry, O. (1997) *Supervising the PhD: a Guide to Success.* Society for Research into Higher Education & Open University Press, Buckingham.

Graham, A. & Grant, B. (1993) *Postgraduate Supervision: Guidelines for Discussion.* Higher Education Research Office, University of Auckland.

Hockey, J. (1995) Getting too close: a problem and possible solution in social science PhD supervision. *British Journal of Guidance and Counselling* 23(2), 199–210.

Murray, R. (1996) Research supervision. *UCoSDA Briefing Paper*, July.

Sheehan, J. (1993) Issues in the supervision of postgraduate research students in nursing. *Journal of Advanced Nursing* 18, 880–885.

Zuber-Skerrit, O. (ed.) (1992) *Starting Research Supervision and Training.* Tertiary Education Institute, Brisbane.

Chapter 4

Selecting a Research Topic and Methodology

Choosing the research topic

When starting to search for an appropriate place to enrol, you are likely to have some idea of the research topic you wish to investigate (if you don't, you should have!). A research topic refers to the general issue to be examined or explored. In the health and social care arena, the topic will usually be rooted in:

(1) A problem or critical incident experienced in practice.
(2) A professional issue which has interested or puzzled the potential researcher.
(3) Issues which emerge from the professional literature or from attending a conference.
(4) Research suggested by supervisors in an area with which they are themselves involved.
(5) An issue which has emerged from previous academic study.
(6) Interest stimulated by personal knowledge or experience.

Sometimes an advertisement in a newspaper or professional journal invites applications for a researcher or research assistant who will enrol for a research degree. In this case you will not be able to choose your own area of research, but will make a personal contribution to a field of investigation for which funding is available. Sometimes an eminent researcher investigates an area significant for the future health and well-being of a large section of the population and invites individuals to work with him or her. This type of research is usually headed by a professor who has special expertise in the field and who supervises several students involved in examining particular and specific problems in his or her area of research. The latter type of study will often, though not always, be laboratory based or situated in the biomedical area.

In such cases, it is wise to check on the freedom to select the focus of study or methodology – a PhD requires room for creativity and innovation. Be sure that the topic will sustain your motivation for a prolonged period. It is also wise to check the duration of funding. Where this is less than the time to MPhil or PhD, you should enquire how the remaining period of study might be financed.

The majority of research students in health and social care will select their own topic and location for study, although this would usually match with departmental interests and areas of research. The problem might be linked to practice, clinical area, educational or other setting in which the student has been involved. Observing or evaluating existing practice might stimulate interest in a particular problem for which research could advance professional knowledge and help patients or clients. Many researchers in the health and social care fields are interested in the outcomes of treatment or care. This is a small sample of the types of question that might be asked, although the research will go much further and include a theoretical framework:

- How do clients benefit from the treatment or care?
- What happens to patients when they have completed their treatment or leave the institution?
- What problems do clients and carers experience during care delivery? How might care be improved?
- What coping strategies do clients adopt, and how successful are they?

You might have encountered the problem in practice, or read about it in a journal article or book and feel that it is important and of interest. Often it emerges naturally in your own setting. On the other hand, a conference topic might stimulate an interest or desire to study a similar issue in a different way.

Example

John works in a drug clinic with young people who regularly use dangerous drugs. He does not know much about their motives or the origin of their problem. The discovery of this knowledge, he feels, might teach him and other care workers to gain a deeper understanding of the young people with whom he works, and possibly help them to overcome the problem.

Professional and occupational issues might include occupational roles, or the policies of the organisation or professional body in which you are located.

Example

Sue, a senior manager in the local social services, wanted to study the issue of homelessness. During her initial literature review she had become interested in the historical perspective and will now investigate the various strategies adopted in the nineteenth and twentieth centuries to cope with this problem, and the underlying ideologies underpinning them.

If you work in the field of education you might wish to investigate teaching and learning strategies to meet the changing needs of clients or services, or the relationship between theory and practice, or find out about the long-term employment prospects of your students.

Example

Moira was interested in studying student nurse placements in the community so that the university could provide large numbers of students with a better experience without overloading community staff. During her initial literature search she discovered some innovations that had been published but not properly evaluated. She decided to use an action research framework to study the impact of introducing these ideas into her own educational setting.

At the point when you first seek academic advice, the research topic is commonly wide in scope but lacks clear focus. It may just consist of a list of questions that you would like to investigate or answer. In fact, many academics prefer this, because it provides an opportunity for finding common ground between themselves and you, the student. They are able to ensure that a suitable methodology is chosen and the study will be appropriate for an MPhil or PhD. Key issues for the initial brainstorming session between you and supervisor might include:

- The topic must excite you and enthuse the supervisor.
- The topic must be researchable.
- You and your supervisor must agree what is to be the main research question.
- The research must be feasible within the available time and resources.
- You and your supervisor should be able to agree an appropriate methodological approach.
- The issue to be studied is worthwhile for a major research project rather than merely a problem for a small study.

If, after the first meetings, you and your supervisor show no sign of reaching agreement on these important issues, it is probably worthwhile seeking advice elsewhere.

Interest and motivation

First and foremost, you must be interested and enthusiastic about your research topic. This will motivate you through the times when you may feel frustrated and discouraged. Taking on research into an area of importance without full commitment is not only unethical, but can lead to boredom and failure to complete. It helps if the supervisor shares your enthusiasm for the chosen topic. Although supervisors' suggestions and guidance should be taken into account, you should resist attempts to be pushed into a specific direction when you lack interest in this area. There is no way, however, in which you can study everything in your area of interest.

Part-time students are frequently motivated by some aspect of personal experience. For example, someone who has had agoraphobia may be highly motivated to study this topic. However, Rudestam and Newton (1992) warn students not to study an area in which they are too involved emotionally, however interesting it may be. It can be difficult to approach the topic in an unbiased way and the research may raise painful issues unforeseen at the outset. A research degree is not the appropriate arena to solve personal problems or to adopt a missionary stance to changing the world.

Researchability of the research question

The research question (Cormack and Benton, 1996) also call it the statement/topic/subject/hypothesis/problem) arises directly from the field. It is a general question about the area to be researched.

The question should, first of all, be researchable. You might wish to address issues which, though important, cannot be researched. Philosophical or moral questions, for instance, might be debated, but they are not easily subjected to empirical research unless you wish to examine the perspectives of clients or professionals on these issues.

It is common for research students in the field of health and social care to want to solve complex problems of service delivery or client care. It is worth noting that MPhil research can address only a small component of this type of problem, while most research to PhD is concerned with ensuring that the right questions are asked and clarifying what the key issues are, rather than coming up with practical solutions.

Feasibility

The question should not only be answerable, but the research must also be feasible within the available time and resources. A lone research student with a fixed-term contract of three years, or part-time PhD student with a limit of five years, must aim to complete the work in the time available. Researchers are often overambitious and find, during the course of their study, that the topic cannot be covered because it is too broad, access to participants is too difficult, or the criteria for sampling are inappropriate to allow completion in time. An experienced supervisor will recognise this at an early stage.

Example

Georgina, a general practitioner (GP) enrolled for a PhD, intended to compare the ways that GPs manage a chronic condition (diabetes) and an acute condition (myocardial infarction). She also wanted to study patient responses and experiences and community nurses' perspectives on the treatment. In early discussions with her supervisor, she realised that the breadth of the research would take her well beyond the allotted time span.

Some researchers require resources which are not readily available or are too expensive to purchase. Even standardised questionnaires, such as those which measure emotional state or quality of life, can be very expensive to obtain if owned by a publishing firm or agency.

Example

Tom wanted to study stress in social workers and his original idea depended on obtaining physiological as well as psychological and behavioural measures. These included ambulant monitoring of blood pressure and heart rate and regular blood tests. Following an initial discussion with an academic adviser at his local university, he was referred to a senior academic working in a national centre of excellence in this field of study for advice. This academic had access to the equipment and the questionnaires needed to measure well-being and psychological arousal.

Sometimes access to the necessary number of participants in the allocated time span is likely to be difficult.

Example

Doreen intended to study the feelings and thoughts of accident survivors who had experienced counselling in a particular region of the country. Not only was this research problematic for ethical reasons, but access to enough volunteers also proved impossible.

Delamont *et al.* (1997) add political feasibility to practical feasibility. It would be foolish of you to include an evaluation of the practices of other professionals, such as, for example, studying nurses' perceptions of patient labelling by doctors. It would be unreasonable to believe that such a study could provide unbiased findings, or that the findings could lead to changes in doctors' behaviour. Similarly, an evaluation of the malpractice of colleagues or managers in a work setting would not be politically feasible. This type of research can only be carried out if it has been specifically asked for by the appropriate gatekeepers, and even then would not be appropriate for many research students.

Selecting the research methodology

Many students select their methodological approach before they have decided on the research question. This may be unwise as the research question determines or at least influences the research design. You need to be prepared to change the area or slant of your research, or the methodology, if necessary. There is an expectation that you have some knowledge of a range of methodologies and methods, or you may be asked to acquire this, before attempting to register for your degree. Only on this basis will you be able to examine the chosen methodology in more depth, understand its strengths, problems and limitations and match it with the research question. Nevertheless, it is important that the chosen methodology should suit your style and fit in with the expertise and preferences of available supervisors. In discussion with you, the first supervisor as main adviser will help you select the appropriate methodology.

The choice of an appropriate research methodology is essential as the validity of the outcomes depends upon it. Methodology refers to the overall approach used to answer the research question and requires philosophical, theoretical and technical justification. The term *method* refers more specifically to the procedures and techniques adopted, for instance the data collection, analysis and sampling processes.

The choice of methodology is linked to the following:

- The research problem and aim of the research
- The subject or discipline
- The world view and style of the researcher
- Practical considerations

Research texts identify two major perspectives in research: quantitative and qualitative, each of which includes a variety of different research methods (Cresswell, 1994; 1998; Bowling, 1997). These are sometimes called *paradigms* although the use of this term is open to dispute (see Atkinson, 1995). The perspectives are based on different sets of assumptions about the nature of reality; that is, they depend on different ideologies, theories of knowledge and ways of collecting and analysing data. Ways of writing up the research are also different in these approaches.

Quantitative research involves the collection of primary data which are quantifiable or can be converted to numbers for the purposes of statistical analysis. The aim of quantitative research is usually to establish generalisable explanations and predictions in relation to the phenomenon in question, and usually takes place against the background of a theoretical framework or set of prior assumptions. Qualitative research is generally carried out where little is known about the phenomenon in question, or where the researcher wishes to explore new interpretations to challenge existing explanations. The theoretical framework for qualitative research is not predetermined but develops out of the study. Some of the key differences can be seen in Fig. 4.1 (p. 51).

Bullock *et al.* (1992) argue that qualitative and quantitative research approaches not only 'differ in the methods employed but also in the perception of the problem and the type of data they produce' (p. 85). It is important, however, not to dichotomise these major research perspectives as they co-exist and may complement each other. Indeed, researchers who are usually pragmatic rather than purist often use both in one study (this is termed *methodological triangulation*). The ontological and epistemological debates surrounding these issues are beyond the scope of this book but can be found in most major research texts about health and social care research (some of which are referenced at the end of this chapter). You are encouraged to familiarise yourself with them before you embark on your research.

Problems in the early stages

Below are just a few common problems which students face in the early stages of their research, together with some possible solutions and comments.

Problem 1 – I know, broadly speaking what I am interested in, but I don't know where to start.

Solution

Write out all the questions that you would like to answer during the course of your study. Now rewrite them in priority order. Now see your supervisor and generate a short list of questions in one column with suitable research methods in the other column. Fig. 4.2 may assist you. Now rethink your priorities.

Comment

Do not imagine that you can solve a large-scale problem during the course of your PhD. You may solve one small one, but you are likely to raise more questions than answers. Regard your study as a significant stage in understanding an important issue. Leave something to study further at postdoctoral level!

Problem 2 – I want to use a qualitative approach but my supervisor is pressing me to use quantitative methods. Should I do what he or she says?

Solution

Discuss the issue with others and decide on the best course of action for you. This will be either to: change your research question; change your methodology; or change your supervisor.

Comment

Don't start until you feel entirely comfortable with all three components (topic, method and supervisor). Don't be afraid to change your supervisor if you are unhappy, but preferably find this out before you reach the stage of registration.

Problem 3 – I think I will need to do some fairly complex analyses later in my research but don't know how I will manage these.

Solution

Check with your supervisor that the necessary expertise will be available to assist you and find out if a suitable training programme exists. If possible, find an external supervisor who will be able to help you when the need arises. If necessary, find a training programme elsewhere and make sure that the funding will be available to support you.

Comment

The members of the research committee who assess your research proposal for registration should ensure that you have all of the support you will need to complete your research. They can block your application if this is not the case

Fig. 4.1 Differentiation between qualitative and quantitative research (adapted from Holloway & Wheeler, 1996).

	Qualitative research	Quantitative research
Aim	Exploration of participants' meaning Understanding, generation of theory from data	Search for explanations Testing hypothesis, prediction, control
Approach	Broad focus Process oriented Context-bound, mostly natural setting Getting close to the data	Narrow focus Product oriented Context-free, often in artificial setting
Sample	Participants, informants Sampling units such as place, time and concepts Flexible sampling which develops during research	Respondents, participants (the term subjects is now discouraged in the social sciences) Sample frame fixed before research starts
Data collection	In-depth, non-standardised interviews Participant observation/fieldwork Documents, photographs, videos	Questionnaire, standardised interviews Tightly structured observation Documents Randomised controlled trials

Contd.

Fig. 4.1 *Contd.*

	Qualitative research	Quantitative research
Analysis	Thematic, latent content analysis Grounded theory, ethnographic analysis, etc.	Statistical analysis
Outcome	A story, an ethnography, a theory	Measurable results
Relationships	Direct involvement of researcher Research relationship close	Limited involvement of researcher Research relationship distant
Rigour	Trustworthiness, authenticity Typicality and transferability	Internal/external validity, reliability Generalisability

Fig. 4.2 Selecting an appropriate methodological stance.

Purpose of study	Methodological approaches	Potential problems
Investigate/describe/understand the nature and meaning of human experience	Qualitative interviewing using: phenomenology, grounded theory, narrative analysis, discourse analysis	Interview technique Ethical issues Detailed analytical procedure
Investigate/describe/understand human experience, behaviour and interaction in a social context	Participant/non-participant observation, and interviewing using: grounded theory ethnography, discourse/conversation analysis	Difficult access, data collection and analysis Ethical issues
Explore context, initiate and evaluate change in a social environment	Action research (incorporating mainly qualitative methods)	Researcher must be a change agent
Describe/compare group attitudes, beliefs, knowledge, self-reported behaviour	Questionnaire surveys using: scaling methods correlation/regression/variance analyses	Detailed preparation, pilot study essential Response rate problems Multivariate analyses

Contd.

Fig. 4.2 *Contd.*

Purpose of study	Methodological approaches	Potential problems
Analyse specific aspects of human behaviour in a particular context	Non-participant recorded observation Documentary analysis Case study design (incorporating qualitative and/or quantitative methods) Diary-keeping/longitudinal measurement using: time series analysis, single case research design	Access Ethical issues Researcher role and identity Specification error Compliance
Evaluate an intervention	Experimental and quasi-experimental designs including randomised controlled trials Qualitative evaluation methods	Ethical issues Field organisation Group allocation Control over variables
Examine an issue from different perspectives	Methodological or sampling triangulation	Organisation Time scale

References

Atkinson, P. (1995) Some perils of paradigms. *Qualitative Health Research* 5 (1), 117–124.

Bowling, A. (1997) *Research Methods in Health: Investigating Health and Health Services*. Open University Press, Buckingham.

Bullock, R., Little, M. & Millhan, S. (1992) The relationship between quantitative and qualitative in social policy research. In *Mixing Methods: Qualitative and Quantitative Research* (ed. J. Brannen), pp. 82–99. Avebury, Aldershot.

Cormack, D.F.S. & Benton, D.C. (1996) Asking the research question. In *The Research Process in Nursing* (ed. D.F.C. Cormack), 3rd edn, pp. 53–63. Blackwell Science, Oxford.

Cresswell, J.W. (1994) *Research Design: Qualitative and Quantitative Approaches*. Sage, Thousand Oaks, CA.

Cresswell, J.W. (1998) *Qualitative Inquiry and Research Design: Choosing Among Five Traditions*. Sage, Thousand Oaks, CA.

Delamont, S., Atkinson, P. & Parry, O. (1997) *Supervising the PhD: a Guide to Success*. Society for Research into Higher Education & Open University Press, Buckingham.

Holloway, I. & Wheeler, S. (1996) *Qualitative Research for Nurses*. Blackwell Science, Oxford.

Rudestam, K.C. & Newton, R.R. (1992) *Surviving your Dissertation: a Comprehensive Guide to Content and Process*. Sage, Newbury Park, CA.

A book such as this is not the place to find a bibliography on research methodologies. The range of texts at different academic levels, currently available, is vast. However, we would advise that, while new postgraduate students may find undergraduate textbooks very helpful in understanding new methodologies, it is necessary to advance from these. External examiners are unlikely to be impressed with references to a limited range of low-level material.

Chapter 5

The Importance of Ethical Issues

The significance of ethical issues

All researchers have to adhere to ethical principles in their research, but in health and social care these are of paramount importance because of close involvement with people who may be in crisis or at a stage in which they are particularly vulnerable. Ethical principles and rules which affirm the rights of participants are not just considered at the start of a study but are revisited throughout the research process and writing up. All good PhD and MPhil theses include a section on relevant ethical issues and how these have been addressed.

Moral principles and ethical guidelines have always existed, though they have changed depending on place and time. They were not, however, fully and systematically formulated for a modern age until the Nuremberg Code (1946), an international code of ethics to govern the conduct of medical research. This was written as a result of unethical medical experiments on non-voluntary participants in Germany during the time of Hitler. The Declaration of Helsinki (1964, revised 1975), published by the World Medical Association and based on the Nuremberg Code, was eventually formulated as an international code of ethics to regulate medical research and forms the basis of many ethical codes.

Sieber (1992) demonstrated that most professional codes of ethics contain common features concerning access to and protection of participants, issues of rights and responsibilities which include privacy and confidentiality, protection of the reputation of the profession, as well as sensitivity and honesty in reporting.

Ethical principles and rules

Beauchamp and Childress (1994) outline four major principles for ethical behaviour which can be applied to research.

(1) Respect for autonomy (independence and self-determination)
(2) Non-maleficence (doing no harm)
(3) Beneficence (doing good)
(4) Justice (fair treatment)

Ethical rules such as veracity, fidelity, privacy and confidentiality are based on these principles.

Autonomy

The right to autonomy means that people's right to self-determination and free, independent choice must be respected. People must have the right to refuse to participate in a study and to withdraw from it at any time if they so wish. Beauchamp and Childress (1994) included rules of privacy and confidentiality. Privacy refers to the treatment of the person and implies that researchers will not attempt to manipulate participants into disclosing issues which they want to keep to themselves. Confidentiality refers to the treatment of the data and implies that the researcher does not disclose issues or ideas that the respondent wishes to keep confidential. As Sieber (1992) states, 'Confidentiality refers to agreements with persons about what may be done with their data' (p. 52). The issue of confidentiality is also important with respect to data taken from confidential documents, such as medical and social work records or letters of complaint, etc. If you are given access to these, you have to keep the identities of individuals strictly confidential so that there is no chance that they can be recognised or connected with the documents.

Confidentiality may be maintained through:

- The use of pseudonyms which only you should be able to match with real names through a code-breaker kept separately.
- Changing names of locations and institutions.
- Changing minor details in the description of participants, if necessary (see Archbold, 1986).
- Changing demographic factors that are unimportant to the research findings.
- Protecting data through the application of codes or numbers, not names.
- Keeping tapes, lists, scripts, etc., secure.

Example

Irene, a clinical psychologist, studied individual cases to identify the effect of a particular treatment. She changed the participants' ages by a few years when drawing a table of respondents. She reported in her findings that she had made minor changes and gave reasons for doing so, but did not reveal the exact detail.

It is never necessary to record the name or location of the research study in the thesis or publications (remember also to delete offending details from letters in the appendices). What is important is the type of organisation and location. Thus the 'Josephine Bloggs Home for the Pusillanimous in Upmarket' might be described as 'A residential home for the fainthearted in an affluent city in the UK'.

Tapes, notes, transcripts or respondent lists are kept secure and should not be labelled with names. Typists who might have access to confidential information (for example, during transcribing) must be reminded that it is unethical and illegal to disclose any of the content. Personal data held on computer are subject to the Data Protection Act and the official responsible within the university must be informed (the ethics committee will ask for confirmation that this has been done).

People who cannot take complete responsibility for their own decisions need special protection. Vulnerable groups include children; those who are frail, confused or seriously ill; those with certain mental health problems and severe learning disabilities. Every effort should be made to communicate the nature of the study to them in a way that they can comprehend and their well-being must be checked at every stage of the research process. Permission should be obtained from parents or legal guardians in the case of those aged under 18. In the case of adults (even those with mental illness or a learning disability), it may be morally advisable to check with close relatives before proceeding, though they are not entitled to give legal consent on behalf of the participant. Timing is an important issue. It would clearly be unethical to attempt to obtain consent just before or after a major operation or during and immediately after a crisis.

Free and independent consent to research may be constrained intentionally or unwittingly by:

- *Lack of information.* There may be a difference between the information given and the information understood. The onus is on you to check that it is fully understood.

- *Social pressures.* Participants may see it as a duty to help others with the same condition or in a similar position, particularly if confronted by you or someone acting on your behalf.

- *Coercion.* Participants may not dare to object for fear that their treatment, or that of someone for whom they are caring, might be adversely affected by their refusal, or that they might be labelled 'difficult' if they refuse to take part.

Example

Sue decided to evaluate a counselling service recently established in her GP practice partnership for travellers. She decided to extend the study for MPhil with the aim of examining travellers' needs and perspectives on the services available to them. Her attention was drawn to the fact that her own patients might report only positive views for fear of losing the service, or because they might be seen as ungrateful. It was therefore thought better if Sue were to study similar services elsewhere. The problem with this was that she specifically wanted to evaluate counselling outcomes in her own locality.

The above example highlights the conflict that can arise between the wants of the individual researcher and needs of the service on one hand, and demands for academic rigour on the other. Archbold (1986) argued that professionals should not do research in their own setting. However, this advice is difficult to follow if you wish to evaluate or explore a problem in your own specific work area (Holloway & Wheeler, 1996). Participants in the research process do not always understand your role as researcher and may see you primarily as a professional to whom they defer or owe loyalty. They need to be assured that their role or contribution is valued in its own right and that their rights to participate or not are fully respected.

Covert research in relation to health and social care presents ethical dilemmas and should not be attempted by MPhil and PhD students. Observation studies are particularly difficult to manage in terms of gaining informed consent from all likely to participate. In a sense, the whole purpose of this type of study is to catch people off their guard. It is probably best to inform all concerned in writing, and through meetings and discussion, before the study begins and by posting prominent notices if the study is to take place in a public area. The advent of closed circuit television (CCTV) has made it easier for people to accept the use of video cameras, but it is essential that you and your supervisor decide what to do should the film reveal unprofessional or even illegal behaviour. In most instances, these issues take priority over the research and must be dealt with even if this means jeopardising the study.

A relatively common occurrence in health and social care research is that a participant will reveal information which you feel, in your professional capacity, should be passed on to other health or social care workers or another agency; for example, a participant expresses suicidal thoughts or complains about the care given by a nurse. Normally, the participants must be asked if they agree to this information being passed on. If they refuse, they should be given details of how to obtain advice and support and asked if they would like someone to contact them. The participants' wishes must be respected unless they were warned, in advance, that information of this sort would be divulged. Participants must be treated as autonomous, and all undertakings of confidentiality must be respected. On the other hand, if maltreatment was actually observed at first hand, this would certainly have to be reported.

Non-maleficence

The principle of *non-maleficence* means that you have a responsibility to ensure that no harm comes to the people you study, and that you do not expose them to any unnecessary risks, be they physical or emotional. This includes looking after the safety of equipment, monitoring ethical processes and debriefing participants (Homan, 1991). You must explain all potential risks to the participants. Danger of physical risk is probably higher in experimental or quasi-experimental research where new treatments could have unforeseen side-effects. Equally, in-depth interviews on sensitive issues or topics could cause emotional damage in certain circumstances.

Example

Bernie, a psychiatric nurse, investigated the effects of suicide on relatives and friends of people who had killed themselves. Many

---

Contd.

times, when interviewing volunteers in his study, he found that they became distressed. He felt guilty about this. He always took the necessary steps to ensure that they felt better before he left, and that they knew where they could obtain help and support. But Bernie was also aware that he fulfilled a useful role in allowing participants to talk at length about their painful experiences, often for the first time. Some wrote to him afterwards to thank him. Although the purpose of the interview was to collect information, it also appeared to have therapeutic value for the participants.

Much has been written on the topic of researching sensitive issues (see Lee 1993; Renzetti & Lee, 1993). If you intend to interview participants in depth on any topic which could cause distress, you should prepare yourself adequately, in advance, to deal with it. Students often state that they will terminate the interview if the participant becomes distressed, but this can leave a feeling of guilt at letting the researcher down. Better to switch the tape recorder off, sit quietly, give verbal reassurance and signal non-verbal reassurance until the individual has talked through their problem or regained their composure. Then ask if they would like to continue with the interview or leave it there. Most prefer to continue.

Adherence to ethical principles and rules is required in relation to research with colleagues as well as clients.

Example

Ken cares for people in a day centre for people with learning disabilities. He wishes to undertake a video observation study of their treatment and care while attending the centre. Ken, his supervisor and the departmental ethics committee, while seeing the advantages of this approach, entered into a long debate about how to obtain informed consent from all concerned and also what might happen should the tape reveal unfavourable findings with respect to staff practices.

Finally, there can be a risk to the well-being of participants if you change the data to suit your own purpose, or suppress information. Participants finding this in the thesis, or a report, book or article, may feel that they have been badly let down.

Beneficence

The principle of *beneficence* implies that the research will ultimately help the individual or the wider society. Any benefits should be balanced against potential harm and must outweigh any risks. Ethics committees are sometimes reluctant to approve research which is seen primarily as serving the training needs or curiosity of the researcher if there is no evidence of direct benefits to respondents, organisation, service delivery or health or welfare in general. The likely beneficial outcomes should be made explicit in applications for grants or ethical approval.

Justice

The principle of *justice* means that participants are treated fairly, that resources are distributed equally and that all research procedures are just and fair to the individuals who take part. Numerous examples exist where a particular medicine or treatment has been withheld from one group and given to another for the purposes of comparison. This should only happen where no evidence already exists to demonstrate that one treatment is actually better than the other. However, there have been examples cited in the media where participants in randomised controlled trials have sued the research sponsor because they felt they were denied access to treatment which, they felt, would have been beneficial to them.

Veracity and fidelity

An open and honest approach is essential to protect the participant and researcher. Indeed, Beauchamp and Childress (1994) identified two additional important ethical rules for all researchers, those of *veracity* (truth telling) and *fidelity* (promise keeping). Veracity means that researchers give true and accurate information to participants in the research and do not mislead them. This is particularly problematic in the case of randomised controlled trials where the therapist is aware that one treatment might be more beneficial than the other. Fidelity demands that any promises should be kept. This includes giving feedback on findings. You need to be aware that finding time at the end of an MPhil or PhD study to return to the participants can be difficult. It may be best to be honest with them about this at the outset, particularly where a large sample is involved.

Examples of unethical studies

Apart from the horrifying experiments of the Nazis during their reign in Germany, the most famous research demonstrating neglect of ethical guidelines are the Tuskegee and Willowbrook studies in the USA.

The Tuskegee study consisted of research into the natural history of syphilis. It started before World War II and carried on until the 1970s when the disease was curable, but no treatment was given so as not to interfere with the research. This was, of course, completely unacceptable (the study also had racist overtones as most of the participants in the study were black).

Willowbrook was a hospital for mentally disabled children. Parents gave consent for their children to be injected with a hepatitis virus because they were promised priority of residential care for their children.

Example of an ethical dilemma and a solution

A researcher wished to evaluate the effects on well-being of an intervention aimed at empowering disabled people in the community, compared to a control group who received standard care. Randomisation to treatment groups was excluded as it seemed unethical for close neighbours to be offered different types of care. Therefore the intervention was offered only in town A and the control group selected from town B. Full information about the study meant that all participants had to know what they were getting or not getting. So that those in town B should not feel deprived, they were advised that the intervention would be made available to them, regardless of participation, if it proved successful in town A (additional money was set aside for this purpose). The response rate in both towns was actually very high, though the findings of the quasi-experiment were not as definitive as those from a randomised controlled trial. The intervention received a mixed response, but the research team kept their promise and offered disabled people in town B the opportunity to receive the intervention if they wished.

Obtaining informed consent

One of the most important ethical principles is that of voluntary, informed consent. In most instances, written consent is essential for the protection of the researcher, university and participants and the consent form is a central feature of this process.

It is essential that the consent form is clearly expressed in ordinary language without jargon. The following list includes some basic components of informed consent:

(1) Provision of name, credentials and a contact address as well as the identity of the funding agency (if there is one).
(2) An explanation of the aims and reasons for the study, including the likely benefits of doing the study.
(3) Outline of the method of data collection, what is expected of them, and the likely timing.
(4) Description of any potential risks anticipated.
(5) Assurance that participation is voluntary and that participants are free to withdraw at any time from the research process.
(6) Promise of anonymity and confidentiality, including a description of how the data will be disposed of at the end of the study.
(7) Promise to answer any questions that participants have about the research.
(8) Reassurance that ongoing treatment will not be affected by the research.
(9) A simple tear-off statement that the individual agrees to take part in the research.

An example of a consent form is given in Fig. 5.1. Students often appear to believe that research is, of necessity, a formal academic process and that letters to participants should reflect this. However, the example given is deliberately phrased in a conversational way to indicate the manner in which the research is likely to be conducted. It contains all the relevant detail but helps to put participants at their ease.

Full informed consent is not once and forever permission, but an ongoing process (Ford & Reutter, 1990). When making the telephone appointment and at the start of the interview, you should restate the purpose of the research, describe the method to be used and make people aware of any potential risks and benefits so they can make a free choice. This may be more difficult in health and social care if the research is social rather than biomedical. Although potentially more

Figure 5.1 Consent form.

Department
University
Address
Telephone

Dear XY (title and name),

Re: People's experiences of counselling in doctors' surgeries
I am an occupational therapist who is currently studying people's
experiences of counselling for my research degree. I understand from
your doctor that you have spoken to a counsellor at some time in the last
six months and wonder if you would mind sharing your experiences with
me.

I do not necessarily wish to know the full details of any personal
problems you may have had, but I am interested to know your feelings
about the service on offer. I do not have a specific list of questions to
ask, but would like you to describe your experience of seeing the
counsellor in your own words. I anticipate that this will take up to an
hour, depending on how much you have to tell.

I would like to tape-record our conversation so that I do not miss
important details. Everything that you say will be treated in the strictest
confidence. Your name and details will not appear in the research, the
tapes will be destroyed after use, and no information will be passed to
any other person or agency without your expressed consent. The
interview may take place in your home or in an office at the university,
whichever you prefer.

If your are willing to talk to me, please return the attached consent form
giving your name, address and telephone number so that I can contact
you to make an appointment. If you would like further information please
contact me on the telephone number at the top of this page. Please do
not feel any pressure to participate – I fully understand if you prefer not
to and your decision will not in any way affect your future treatment or
care.

Thank you for reading this letter. I look forward to meeting you in due
course, should you decide to accept this invitation.

Yours sincerely,

Jane Gray
Research student

Contd.

Consent form: People's experiences of counselling in doctors' surgeries

I am quite happy for Jane Gray to interview me about my experiences of counselling.

I understand that everything I say will be treated in the strictest confidence, that I am completely free to withdraw from the study at any time I choose without any need for explanation, and that such a decision will not affect any aspect of my future treatment or care.

NAME (please print)

SIGNATURE

ADDRESS

TELEPHONE NUMBER:

The best time to contact me is:

---

risky, biomedical research is less ambiguous and the risks can be more easily identified. Qualitative researchers have particular problems with informed consent, and the need to warn participants that an interview might precipitate distress is a contentious issue. Furthermore, since qualitative research focuses on the interpretations of participants, detailed information about the path of the research cannot be fully described before the research starts, as it might guide the participants in a specific direction. Sometimes full information cannot be achieved (Kimmel, 1996), as researchers who are also health and social care professionals may have more knowledge of the research process or the participants' condition than they are able to share.

Negotiating access and managing gatekeepers

Gaining access to organisations

For research within any organisational setting, including obtaining names and details of participants, you need first to approach the *gatekeepers*, those individuals controlling access to the organisation. Gatekeepers are primary decision-makers such as managers, clinical directors and ethics committees, together with their secretaries or administrators. They also include professionals or practitioners who provide a direct link with the participants (for example, in distributing letters of introduction, questionnaires, etc.). Managers are normally first in line with the power to grant, impose conditions on, or withhold, access. A personal approach is often best, but these are busy people. It is a good idea to send them a brief outline of the study, together with copies of letters to participants and ethical consent forms, and then arrange a meeting to explain what you wish to do and how it will benefit the service in the longer term. From their point of view, their first priority is to protect the interests of clients/patients, employees and the organisation. One of the most common reasons for refusal is that too much research is already taking place in the same setting.

You should, prior to any meeting with gatekeepers, consider what course of action to take should the findings prove unfavourable to the organisation in which it is to be located. It is better to consider this possibility at an early stage than to find oneself faced with the problem after the event. Negative findings can also cause problems for publication, especially where it is difficult to protect the location. Similarly, if the research is sponsored by an agency (for example, to test a new form of treatment or care), you should be aware of potential conflicts of interest which might arise and negotiate questions of ownership before the start of the research. Most universities have a policy on intellectual property rights and insist that ownership of data is in their hands, although there may be negotiated exceptions. There are some organisations, such as the Home Office or Ministry of Defence, which can insist on the right to suppress publication of a thesis for a stipulated period of time, in order to protect the national interest. They may also demand to approve any publications which emerge from the findings.

Ethics committees

Permission to conduct any research in health and social care must be obtained from relevant ethics committees. Some university faculties or departments have their own committees. Organisations such as the Home Office have their own committee. Social services departments do not all have ethics committees, in which case permission from the director or senior managers suffices. Application to the local research ethics committee (LREC) applies to all research which involves NHS patients (in hospital, nursing home or community), including obtaining names and addresses from an NHS source, or use of NHS staff time or resources. The application form may be obtained from the secretary to the committee, whose name and address your supervisor might know, or you will be able to obtain the form and local address from the NHSE R&D directorate. The form is accompanied by guidelines which should be adhered to rigorously. You will be asked to append all letters to clients and consent forms and provide the signature of the manager or clinical director concerned. Where the study covers more than one local area, check on the procedure with the NHSE R&D directorate.

At the earliest opportunity, remember to check how often the ethics committee meets and when you are likely to receive a response. Some committees meet regularly, others do not. Some actually postpone meetings until they have sufficient applications to consider. If you do not hear soon after the meeting, check on the outcome and affirm the importance of the decision.

You will need to convince the committee of the benefits that the study will confer in the longer term. You will also need to explain succinctly and justify your methodology. Some LRECs are medically dominated and unfamiliar with qualitative research, in which case you will need to give references to support your methodology. It is common for such a committee to ask to see the interview schedule. If using unstructured interviews, justify and reference your interview technique and give an example of how the interview will begin and be sustained.

Students applying for external research funding are normally required to provide written consent from gatekeepers, including ethics committees, with their research proposal. Students applying to study for the MPhil/PhD are normally required to submit written consent from all gatekeepers, including ethics committees, with their application to register with the university. This provides a safeguard for student, supervisor, university and, where appropriate, the funding agency.

One point frequently raised in applications to LRECs is the need to ask permission from GPs to conduct interviews with patients who have left hospital, even when the interviews are concerned primarily with their hospital treatment. The names and addresses of GPs are generally easy to obtain, and it is probably advisable to inform them as a matter of courtesy, since they may still be involved in treatment. The problem is that they rarely reply. A good tip is to write a letter outlining the study, stating that you intend to interview their patient(s) (state names and details) and on what topic. Then invite them to return a tear-off strip or telephone you if there is any reason why they think that this might *not* be appropriate. If you don't hear from them by the specified date, you can safely proceed. They are sometimes very helpful in informing you of changes of address or recent illness or even death.

It is possible to bypass applications to LRECs by recruiting members of the public direct, for example by advertising or snowballing. However, the research degrees committee of the university will require that you have addressed the full ethical implications of your study in your application to register for a research degree.

Access to participants via practitioners

Once approval for the study has been gained from all the necessary authorities, you have still to obtain the cooperation of practitioners and professionals who act as gatekeepers to participants. Experience suggests that even when individuals agree to help and seem enthusiastic about the study, letters of introduction go astray and questionnaires fail to get delivered, thus reducing the response rate for reasons which cannot be accounted for. The most likely explanation is that the task of delivery gets forgotten because it is outside the daily routine. On the other hand, some practitioners put too much pressure on participants and insist that they sign the consent form there and then. The process of making a telephone appointment prior to further contact provides a safeguard against this type of coercion, as participants can then make up a reasonable excuse not to proceed (often not the real reason). If they do this, do not be tempted to pursue them too hard as this might be construed as harassment.

Accessing participants' personal space

A researcher who enters the home of the participant does so as a guest. This applies equally to those living in residential care accommodation as it does to the home owned by the participant. Even practitioners sometimes forget that a private room in a residential home must not be invaded without the prior consent of the participant. Research which takes place in public rooms of such residences also raises interesting ethical issues and care must be taken not to invade the privacy of other residents. It is polite for researchers to introduce themselves to all concerned on arrival and to ensure that participants and non-participants alike are accorded privacy.

Ending the research relationship

The relationship between researcher and participant does not always end with completion of the study, at least from the point of view of those who have participated. Debriefing can help by giving participants a chance to interact with you, hear about your findings and your explanations and ask questions. You can discuss more fully the potential use of the study and share the knowledge which has been gained. For reasons of time and money, it is inadvisable to promise a copy of the study, but a short summary or brief discussion in a letter of thanks is appreciated by those who give their time and disclose details about themselves.

A cautionary tale

A study by Langer and Rodin (1976) set out to examine the effects of giving more control over volunteer visitors to elderly people in residential care settings. By the end of the study, the group who had control over visits were less depressed and more active than the control group. However, on returning a year later, the research team were shocked to find that the death rate in the experimental group during the intervening period was double that of the control group and those still alive were more depressed (Rodin & Langer, 1977). This research speaks for itself in highlighting some unforeseen effects of interfering in people's lives for the purposes of well-intentioned research.

References

Archbold, P. (1986) Ethical issues in qualitative research. In *From Practice to Grounded Theory: Qualitative Research in Nursing* (eds W.C. Chenitz & J.M. Swanson), pp. 155–163. Addison-Wesley, Menlo Park, CA.

Beauchamp, T.L. & Childress, J.F. (1994) *The Principles of Biomedical Ethics.* Oxford University Press, New York.

Ford, J.S. & Reutter, L.I. (1990) Ethical dilemmas associated with small samples. *Journal of Advanced Nursing* 15, 187–191.

Holloway, I. & Wheeler, S. (1996) *Qualitative Research for Nurses.* Blackwell Science, Oxford.

Homan, R. (1991) *Ethics in Social Research.* Longman, London.

Kimmel, A.J. (1996) *Ethical Issues in Behavioural Research.* Blackwell, Cambridge, MA.

Langer E.J. & Rodin, J. (1976) The effects of choice and enhanced personal responsibility for the aged: a field experiment in an institutional setting. *Journal of Personality and Social Psychology* 34 (2), 191–198.

Lee, R. (1993) *Doing Research on Sensitive Topics.* Sage, London.

Renzetti, C. & Lee, R. (1993) *Researching Sensitive Topics.* Sage, Newbury Park, CA.

Rodin, J. & Langer, E.J. (1977) Long-term effects of a control-relevant intervention with the institutionalised aged. *Journal of Personality and Social Psychology* 35(12), 897–902.

Sieber, J.E. (1992) *Planning Ethically Responsible Research*. Sage, Newbury Park, CA.

Chapter 6

Reviewing the Literature

Maintaining a bibliography

The first essential task for all postgraduate researchers is to set up a system for the systematic recording of all reference material (Rudestam & Newton, 1992). The moment you start reading *anything* you will need to record the following minimum information:

- Author's surname and initials
- Date of publication
- Title of article/book chapter
- Full journal title, volume number, issue number and page numbers
- Full book title
- Location and name of publisher
- Page numbers of book chapters or direct quotations
- The library or other source from which the book was obtained (so that you can retrieve it at a later date)

The method of recording is a matter of personal preference. Some students develop a card system, others a computer file or bibliographic relational database such as *ProCite* or *Reference Manager* in which they detail the references and summarise the associated literature. Detailed notes tend to be useful, particularly when they provide summaries of articles or chapters in books. We have both lost useful references because of inadequate note taking. When you wish to remember a pithy quote or a list of ideas, make sure to add the page number to the reference of the relevant book or article. It leads to frustration when you wish to retrieve an idea to have to find or reread a whole book. It is also time-consuming when you have to search for a town or date of publication, or the initials of authors at the completion of the thesis.

It is helpful, as soon as you start writing, to maintain an active reference list which contains all the references you have used or obtained for use in the form they will be presented in the thesis. It may also be useful to maintain a separate list (or separately coded list) of all references which are likely to be needed or have been ordered, so this is with you whenever you need it. Details can be transferred from the 'required' list to the 'active' list as copies are obtained. This produces a complete reference list at each stage of the thesis and saves a huge amount of work at the stage of the final draft.

At the beginning of an MPhil or PhD it is often difficult to judge what is likely to be relevant and what is not. Although the costs are considerable, it can save a lot of trouble in the long term if all potentially useful material is photocopied and filed for future reference. This is particularly important for extracts from books which have been obtained from external libraries or interlibrary loan and may be difficult or expensive to obtain again.

The purpose of the literature review

Carrying out a literature review is a research skill necessary for all researchers. The literature review should demonstrate that students:

- have both broad and specific knowledge about their area of study;
- have understood related theoretical and methodological issues;
- know how to use and acknowledge the work of others, and demonstrate how it informs their own study;
- are able to use and integrate others' work to modify their own.

Describing, criticising and relating are the essential tasks of reviewers (Afolabi, 1992). Describing other writers' work involves summarising its aims, methodology, main findings and conclusions. Critiquing means evaluating published work through showing its strengths and weakness as well as highlighting its significance. It should point to errors (for instance, if an inappropriate methodology was adopted), establish its validity and reliability, and ensure that the conclusions relate to the aims of the research. Familiarity with the literature will prevent you from replicating the flaws and weaknesses of other research studies. An element of critical analysis is always part of a literature review.

Bruce (1994) suggests that the literature review can be seen in terms of 'process and product' (p. 218). The process has a number of stages: it is used to establish and justify the research question and identify the gap in relevant knowledge. Familiarity with other work in your area of interest enables you to avoid unnecessary repetition and thereby 'reinventing the wheel'. You can later compare the findings of your own research with that of others. The product involves a coherent critique and synthesis of relevant studies.

The stages of the literature review may be summarised as:

(1) *Preliminary review*. This is undertaken during preparation of the research proposal. Its main purpose is to ensure, as far as possible at this stage, that you are building on the work of others and not duplicating it. It will identify key theorists and researchers in the field, together with some of the most seminal and recent studies.

(2) *Main review*. This takes place in the early stages of the research to locate the work in context and provide a comprehensive overview of the subject area, theoretical frameworks, existing research in the field (including PhD theses) and methodologies.

(3) *Updating and review of new areas*. Quite commonly the research reveals new areas for review as the work progresses.

(4) *Review of literature in relation to your own findings*.

(5) *Final updating* prior to submission and viva.

The purpose of the literature review is:

(1) To establish the state of relevant knowledge and theory in the area of study.
(2) To identify key writers in the field.
(3) To evaluate, critically, the findings, conclusions and thought processes of other writers in the area of study.
(4) To justify the research and set boundaries for it in the light of others' findings.
(5) To compare the findings of your study with those of others.
(6) To examine arguments which confirm or contradict your own research and engage in academic debate.

It is inadvisable to neglect a comprehensive review of the literature at an early stage, even when using qualitative methods, because the planned research may have been carried out in a similar form before.

> **Example**
>
> Mary, a GP and part-time MPhil student, had discussed her research area and the research problem with her supervisor, who recommended she should conduct a literature review. Mary disregarded the supervisor's advice because she was highly motivated to start the empirical part of her research and wished to interview patients. Several months into her study she found that she was replicating a piece of research that had been carried out quite recently by a nurse researcher. Mary had then to redirect her study focusing on different issues from those she had originally envisaged.

The first important task is to determine and define the topic and concepts on which to focus. The literature itself will then point to future directions that might be taken.

The literature search

Sources

Articles and books on relevant topic areas can be found by scanning the databases, many of which are computerised, available in the university library, on-line or on CD-ROM. Those undertaking a research degree in the field of health care have the advantage of being able to use libraries based in hospitals as well as those in academic institutions. *To cite all important databases for the literature would go too far for a book like this, but we will mention a few relevant sources for the literature review.* Some useful databases include:

- **Medline** – the bibliographic database of the US National Library of Medicine which contains articles in international journals in the medical field, such as in primary health care, the neurosciences, environmental and public health, health informatics etc.
- **Citation Index for Nursing and Allied Health** (CINAHL) – the bibliographic database for nursing and allied health professions. Through this you can find details of articles in English language nursing and biomedical journals.
- **Care data** – a smaller database about social and community care in the UK.
- **Midirs** – the midwifery digest.

- **Cochrane and York databases** for identifying systematic reviews.
- **Biological abstracts** – these refer to articles in biology and related fields.
- **PsycLIT** – psychological abstracts of articles (and books from 1987) from the American Psychological Association.
- **Sociofile** – articles in the field of sociology, social policy and related studies.
- **Qualidata** is an archival resource centre for qualitative research.
- The **Social Science Citation Index** includes articles from 14 000 journals across social science disciplines.

Many UK universities subscribe to the **Bath Information and Data Services** (BIDS). This is available on the Internet and requires a password which the university library will supply free of charge.

Material is increasingly being published on the Internet, either via electronic journals or individual websites. While this has the advantage of being up to date, much of this information is not subjected to peer review and needs to be treated with some caution.

Search methods

For research at this level, the search for key text words, and later key authors, is particularly useful. First enter a generic word (which generates thousands of articles) and then combine with more specific words until the number of articles is reduced to fewer than 100. Scan these to see if they are relevant and correct the search or refine further if necessary. Select those which are relevant and print out the details. Librarians are generally very helpful, and university librarians offer special sessions to help research students learn to search databases. Some organisations (such as the Royal College of Nursing) will conduct a search for you, but this is unlikely to be adequate for research at this level.

Collecting articles and books

The library is unlikely to stock all of the books and journals necessary for research at this level. Much material of potential interest may be found in obscure or foreign sources. The interlibrary loan system is designed for the purposes of locating such material, either from other institutions or from the British Library. PhD theses are usually supplied on microfiche which can be read on a machine in the library. The interlibrary loan system is normally quite quick (about one to two weeks) and in most cases university libraries make no charge. However, you should be aware that it costs about £6 (at 1998 prices) to obtain a photocopy of one article from this source. If you have access to NHS libraries, you are well advised to make use of the regional library networks to obtain the books and articles available in participating libraries. It is sometimes useful, and quicker, to make a visit to libraries at other universities if they have relevant specialist material. Most university libraries offer open access to enable reading and photocopying although some, including London University, do this only when their own students are down for the vacation. Alumni may be able to apply for lending rights at their old university and this may apply to practitioner diplomates as well as graduates. Some universities will grant lending rights to research students from other universities on payment of a small annual fee, enabling students studying at a distance to gain access to local facilities.

Exhausting the search

Electronic databases will not provide an exhaustive search. For the PhD, in particular, it is necessary to follow references well back in time to ensure that you can trace the development of key concepts and identify seminal theorists. These often predate articles entered on the current databases. Therefore it is necessary to follow up relevant references from material you have already acquired. You will know that the search is becoming exhausted when few or no new references appear.

Personal contact is a useful way of finding out what research is currently taking place in the field. Access to universities through the Internet identifies research groups and staff lists with research interests and e-mail addresses for follow-up. E-mail is often the best means of communication with all academics since it allows them to read the message and respond at their leisure. Other researchers, even senior academics, are normally delighted to discuss their work with you and offer advice. Those who do not respond may just be extremely busy or could be on sabbatical leave (normally up to six months).

Key aspects of the main literature review

The main literature search should be sufficiently comprehensive to locate all relevant material, but cannot be all-inclusive. The search may initially be broad but should become progressively more focused. Not all of the material identified in the literature search will be used in the literature review. While searching for particular concepts you will often find too many to retrieve and critique. This means that the research topic and/or the search may be too broad and has to be refined. Frank (1996) suggests that a comprehensive search will uncover too many books and articles. The student should, so she says, 'search backwards from the latest information available' (p. 68). It is more important for the literature to be representative rather than all-inclusive. It is acceptable in some circumstances to present an overview of previous studies in tabular form, identifying the methods and research instruments used, the key findings and any other salient aspects.

The literature review should be up to date. Too few up-to-date references indicates a lack of effort on the part of the student. The latest work related to all aspects of the study should be debated. This means ongoing searches for connected research and identification of current thinking about the field of research, right up to the point at which candidates submit their theses. Although you will be selective in your choice and up to date, don't forget to discuss classic and seminal studies which have influenced the whole field.

The review must be systematic. Organisation can be achieved through the use of headings and subheadings. Ideas can be regrouped as the study goes on. The literature may be grouped chronologically or conceptually. Occasionally students list and critique a series of seemingly unrelated studies and neglect to give a coherent synthesis.

Defining the boundaries of the literature review

Sometimes researchers fail to find any literature in the field of study. This may have two reasons.

(1) There is no literature in the topic area. This demonstrates a real need for the research.
(2) The initial search was inadequate and needs to be redefined (for example, to include relevant theoretical or methodological perspectives from closely related topics).

Example

Jack Burgess is carrying out a study on the way physiotherapy tutors learn their roles. He has just started an initial literature

Contd.

review which consists of a number of sections. In section one, he wished to discuss studies of socialisation and role learning in physiotherapy teaching, but he cannot find any research studies or literature. This tells him that his research is an important piece of work giving him an opportunity to advance knowledge in his field of study (or it might tell the reader of the proposal that he has not carried out an adequate search). Further searches lead to the literature on teacher socialisation which opens up ideas for Jack's own research. The literature on theories of socialisation also yields useful material.

The preliminary literature review (for the research proposal) should consist of the main pertinent studies, including classic and most recent research as well as the methodological approaches and procedures used for them. Gaps in current knowledge become apparent at this point. By the end of this review, the reader should be in no doubt that a particular study, in the form described by the researchers, is most appropriate to meet the research aim.

Personal experiences in practice normally help you to justify the area of interest. You may look, in the first instance, at the literature in the fields of health or social care. But a review of the literature for a higher degree should extend into related disciplines where appropriate. For example, a study of stress in nursing might include a review of material from business and health service management, organisational or occupational psychology, health psychology, medical sociology and/or psychophysiology, depending on the focus of the topic. Equally, the nursing literature might give doctors a broader view of the type of research methods that they can use, while social workers might investigate the theoretical ideas of psychologists who have touched upon their area of study. It is extremely embarrassing to enter the viva and find that the examiner knows of work from a different discipline which predates or invalidates some of the work that you have done.

Primary and secondary literature sources

A review of the literature at this level consists mainly of a critical review of primary sources from first-hand accounts of research and other original work contained in books, articles, theses and dissertations.

Secondary literature sources, consisting of information summarised or cited in primary sources (for instance, from reviews of research or summaries in articles or books), are not sufficient for postgraduate degrees. Therefore, references such as 'Smith (1984, cited Jones, 1996)' are generally inappropriate in MPhil/PhD work. You should always attempt to examine the original study rather than taking the interpretation – or misinterpretation! – of others. The use of primary sources will often involve obtaining material which is old or out of print, so plenty of time should be allowed for this.

The role of the literature review in quantitative studies

Quantitative studies are normally based on an approach which requires a clear theoretical framework and valid and reliable measurement instruments which are clearly defined and justified. One of the purposes of the literature review is to establish a suitable theoretical framework and identify suitable measures. This will require a critical review of the theories, models and measures which have previously been used in similar types of research or (for PhD) the development of a novel theoretical approach. It is up to you to justify the approach you decide to take, based on a review of the relevant literature.

Health and social care disciplines are starting to develop theories of their own, but often tend to borrow theoretical approaches from other disciplines in the biological or social sciences. It is therefore essential for you to talk to experts from other disciplines in order to gain an initial sense of direction for your search. The theoretical model will determine the nature of the measurement instruments to be used. It is very likely that someone has already developed an instrument to serve a similar purpose. This instrument may be used as it stands, or will require modification (e.g. from American to English). Alternatively, you may decide to develop your own instrument, but you will have to present a very sound case for doing so, based on a critical review of the literature.

The literature review for a quantitative study may be quite extensive and involve several discrete chapters of the thesis.

The role of the literature review in qualitative studies

A qualitative literature review is not as extensive and is sometimes called an 'initial literature review'. Its main purpose is to find out what research has been done before and how it was carried out in order to make a case for the present study. The first step for the researcher is to trawl the relevant and related literature, summarise the main ideas from these studies as well as some of the problems and contradictions found, and show how they relate to the project in hand. The status of previous related studies is critically assessed with particular reference to the methodologies used.

It is not necessary in qualitative reports to review every piece of known research in the field or to give a critical review of all the literature from the very beginning of the thesis. Indeed, some qualitative researchers suggest that there is a danger of being directed by existing research and theoretical frameworks rather than letting the research develop from the perspectives of the participants or generating and developing a theory. Many supervisors prefer that research degree students conducting qualitative studies write up their initial literature review so that they can assess students' writing, critical thinking, debating and presentation skills. We would support this view. However, we also recognise that you may need to relocate much of this work into the discussion of emergent themes as the thesis progresses.

Presenting the literature review

The introduction to the literature review provides the framework which indicates the various areas of research and the time span to which the literature is confined; for instance, apart from seminal work, you might discuss the literature of the last two decades relating to the topic. The main part describes and evaluates the evidence from other studies, puts it in context and synthesises the main available literature. The literature review generally finishes with a conclusion which legitimates your own research.

The literature review might be divided into several sections; for example:

- Background information which shows the need for a study on this topic.
- An overview of research related to the topic area (organised chronologically or conceptually).
- A summary of what is known about the topic area.
- A critical evaluation of the literature directly relevant to the topic, including the methodological approach taken.
- A summary of the key findings from the literature search and evaluation.
- The contribution which your work is likely to make to the field.

Some theses contain a section entitled 'literature review', but it is often better to structure the introductory chapters around the issues in question and incorporate the essential aspects of the literature review into these. In this way, the central argument (or thesis) is more easily developed and conveyed.

Rudestam and Newton (1992) differentiate between background information, descriptive material and studies of direct relevance to the research. Background studies may be described more superficially while more descriptive work demands a more careful critique as it will show the direction of the study. Directly relevant material will be carefully examined and critiqued, because it is of major significance. On the basis of the literature review, you will be able to develop a coherent argument for your own study. At the end of the initial review you will be familiar with the major existing literature related to the work and have established a framework for your own research.

The length of the review

The introductory chapters for a thesis may contain up to 10 000 words, depending on the type of study. Any longer and the examiner will become suspicious that you are unable to focus on essential detail of the research itself. It is obvious that a 40 000 word MPhil does not demand the same extensive literature review as a 70 000- or 80 000-word PhD. Although you must summarise the relevant literature, take a critical stance and make use of the writings of others, you are not necessarily expected to exhaust the literature connected to the study. The literature review which appears in the final thesis may represent only a fraction of the literature originally read or reviewed. Much of this is an important part of the learning process, particularly for PhD. It enables you to present and defend the thesis in a confident and competent way but will not necessarily form part of the thesis.

Example

Stan wanted to study stress in senior hospital managers for his part-time PhD and needed to identify a suitable framework for a national survey. He spent many weeks examining, in detail, a vast literature on different theories of stress and coping and eventually

---

Contd.

rejected all but two as the basis of his study. In writing up his thesis, he gave a detailed critical account of his selected theoretical framework (he actually integrated two theories), but excluded a detailed review of the others. However, his initial thorough search paid off when he was able to respond easily to his external examiner's demands for a more detailed explanation as to why he had rejected other theoretical approaches.

Example

Val set out to study the management of pain associated with fibromyalgia. Her initial search and detailed review extended to definitions of pain, theories of pain, physiology of pain, distinctions between acute and chronic pain, coping with pain, coping theory, treatment approaches to chronic pain and their efficacy, and all this before she had even started to review the literature specific to fibromyalgia and related disorders. Most of this work, though essential to her understanding of fibromyalgia, did not appear in great detail in her thesis.

Continuing the search and review

The initial literature review is complete when the major relevant areas of the research and related theoretical aspects have been discussed and a clear reason for the study has emerged. The literature review does not end with the initial search and critique, but it continues throughout the study, parallel to data collection and analysis. New work might be generated by others at any time. Your own theories and ideas may become more focused during the research and have to be linked to those of other writers. The continued search for related ideas and themes is particularly important for qualitative researchers.

A short guide to the literature review

- Critically examine other people's work in your specific area of study.
- Be as comprehensive as necessary (depending on your approach) but do not include non-essential literature.

- Be up to date but do not forget early seminal work.
- Be systematic.
- Avoid the use of secondary sources.
- Demonstrate the potential contribution of your own research to the topic area.
- Review the literature throughout your research, not only at the initial stages.
- Integrate the literature and relate it to your work.

References

Afolabi, M. (1992) The review of related literature in research. *Journal of Information and Library Research* **4**(1), 56–59.

Bruce, C.S. (1994) Research students' early experiences of the dissertation literature review. *Studies in Higher Education* **19**(2), 217–229.

Frank, S. (1996) Reviewing the literature: use of library and information systems. In *Research Methods: Guidance for Postgraduates* (ed. T. Greenfield), pp. 47–51. Arnold, London.

Rudestam, K.C. & Newton, R.R. (1992) *Surviving your Dissertation: a Comprehensive Guide to Content and Process*. Sage, Newbury Park, CA.

Further Reading

Bruce, C. (1994) Supervising literature reviews. In *Quality in Postgraduate Education* (eds O. Zuber-Skerrit & Y. Ryan), pp. 143–155. Kogan Page, London.

Fink, A. (1998) *Conducting Research Literature Reviews: From Paper to the Internet*. Sage, Thousand Oaks, CA.

Chapter 7

Writing the Proposal

Developing a proposal

The research proposal is a plan of work in which you describe and justify your proposed research programme. There are two distinct types of proposal you need to know about: (1) the proposal which every student must write in order to register with the institution which will eventually give the award of MPhil or PhD; and (2) the proposal which is written in application for a studentship or to attract other research funding. This section focuses predominantly upon (1), although an example of a funding proposal, together with some advice, is given at the end of this chapter.

An academic research proposal must be submitted to the research degrees committee of the faculty or university in order to register for a research degree. Full details of the procedures involved in registration will be found in the student handbook (see Chapter 8). If you register in a college which does not have its own degree-awarding powers, you will find that your proposal must be accepted by the college degrees committee and that of the awarding university, adding substantially to the time required for this process. The proposal enables senior academics who represent the awarding organisation to judge the potential quality and standard of the work and the likelihood that it will ultimately meet the required standard for an MPhil or PhD. They have the power to accept or invite modifications to the proposal. Rarely do they reject it outright.

Some degrees committees include academics from other disciplines. Therefore, the proposal should be written for an informed reviewer who has good general knowledge of research but little specific knowledge of the research field. Avoid the use of jargon and complex terminology, briefly explain practice-related issues, and define or briefly describe concepts related to theory or methodology (without being too wordy). It is a good idea to ask someone from another discipline to read it before submission to identify any words or phrases they don't fully understand.

The purpose of the research proposal is to convince the research degrees committee that:

- The choice of topic is justified and appropriate.
- The aims and objectives are achievable.
- The key issues have been recognised and understood.
- There is a detailed plan of work which meets the stated aims and is achievable.
- The student is adequately prepared, educationally, to conduct the research.
- The proposed research training programme meets the student's needs.
- The resources necessary to bring the study to a successful conclusion are available (for example, access, expenses, library facilities, equipment).
- The supervisory team is sufficiently knowledgeable and experienced to support the student to a successful conclusion.

Most higher education institutions have detailed guidelines for writing proposals, and it is important to follow these. They are subject to variations in the length and detail required. It is the responsibility of the main supervisor or director of studies to ensure that you are educationally prepared and have the resources necessary to undertake the work, although you should be aware that the main reasons why research degrees committees refer back proposals concern the issues listed above. However, your main concern at this early stage of the work is to prepare the plan of investigation.

Supervisors are expected to assist with the writing of the proposal, but you must take ownership of it. We know of instances where supervisors have written the proposal and students have found themselves committed to a plan of work which they eventually sought to change or even abandon. It is better to locate differences in perspective or opinion between you and your supervisors at this early stage than to have to confront them later after a substantial investment in time and resources has already been made.

The purpose of the plan of investigation is to communicate clearly *what* is to be investigated, *why* it is being done, *who* will participate, and *how* and *where* the research will be carried out. The ability to articulate this goes some way to demonstrate that the candidate is competent to do the work. Because committee members often have large numbers of proposals to read and consider, it should be concise and succinct.

The elements of the proposal

The plan of work includes a discussion of the research problem, the justification for doing the research, the location of the research in the context of previous work, the research design and procedures as well as the timetable of the research. It normally consists of the following:

(1) Title of the study
(2) Abstract
(3) Statement of main aim and sub-aims or objectives (distinguishing between those for MPhil and those for PhD, where appropriate)
(4) Rationale
    (a) The statement of the problem
    (b) Background related to practice
    (c) Brief overview of existing literature, identifying key research and theorists (preliminary literature review)
(5) Likely outcomes for practice
(6) Proposed method
    (a) Justification for selection of method
    (b) Procedures for data collection and analysis
    (c) Limitations and delimitations of the research
    (d) Issues of validity and reliability (or their equivalents)
    (e) Ethical considerations
(7) Timetable or timeline to MPhil or PhD

Title

The title is normally provisional and may be expected to change during the course of the research process. Bond (1996) suggests that the title should be broad enough to accommodate possible changes. However, you should check the university regulations, as some institutions demand a permanent title, either at registration or transfer. Often they have to be formally notified of a change of title well before the completion of the thesis. The title should be succinct and not too long, but must accurately reflect the content of the potential study. The title enables other researchers to locate a thesis of relevance to their own studies. Locke *et al.* (1993) advise that the inclusion of terms such as 'a study', 'an analysis', 'aspects of', 'an investigation of' are obsolete. However, subtitles such as 'a survey', 'a grounded theory', 'an ethnography' may be useful as they identify the methodology used in the study. Facetious or cryptic titles are unsuitable for a thesis.

Examples of actual titles

A *nurse-led health education programme for smoking cessation: evaluation using the theory of planned behaviour* (Galvin, 1997. Dr Kathleen Galvin was a nurse who is now departmental research coordinator at a university)

Narrative identity and dementia: narrative and emotion in older people with dementia (Mills, 1995; Dr Marie Mills has a social work background and is now a psychologist and counsellor)

The use of operant conditioning to reinstate the speech of schizophrenic patients (Baker, 1971; Professor Roger Baker is a clinical psychologist who heads a local NHS research and development support unit)

Abstract

The abstract, where required, is a succinct summary (about 150–200 words) of the major elements of the proposal. It states the research problem and aim and describes briefly the design and procedures to be adopted and the potential contribution the project will make to professional practice. It is mostly written in the future tense and should be written in clear, understandable language. It is easier to write the abstract after the rest of the proposal has been completed.

Aim and objectives

The aim of the research is a broad statement of intention to investigate a particular phenomenon. This is usually followed by a sequential list of more specific sub-aims or objectives which are direct steps towards meeting the stated aim. The language of these should match the chosen methodology, so that the reviewers can see that the methods of data collection will address each stated objective and satisfy the overall aim.

Rationale

The rationale for the research contains an explanation and justification for conducting research to address the stated aim. It will be rooted, at least in part, in the researchers' experiences in practice, but also depends on the results of the preliminary literature search. The rationale enables the reviewer to recognise that the area to be examined is important, that the research will contribute to knowledge in the field and has important implications for health or social care or professional practice.

Literature review

The literature review for the proposal is of a preliminary nature, as discussed in Chapter 6. It is the result of an initial search in books and recent articles for key studies which are related and important to the research. You should demonstrate that you are familiar and up to date with recent studies in the field, main researchers, methodologies previously used and relevant theory and theorists. This will enable you to locate your own study in the context of these and demonstrate where your study fills gaps in existing knowledge or research perspectives in the field.

Research design and methods

The research design is a general description of the structural framework of the research. It includes strategies and procedures likely to be followed, including methods of data collection, framework for sampling and approach to data analysis.

The methods selected should be explained and justified. The study population, method of sampling and sampling criteria should be described and justified. It is important to explain how access to the sample will be gained. Research instruments or tools for data collection, where known, should be identified and their purpose stated. Alternatively, the process of instrument identification or development should be described. You must demonstrate how you intend to analyse your data. At this stage, it is best to describe and reference known methods of data collection and analysis.

Where it is anticipated that the research will take place in a series of sequential stages, give details of the initial stage and then illustrate how you anticipate the other stages might develop. Each stage should relate to the stated objectives. It is expected that the research strategies for the PhD will be linked to the development of new knowledge (facts, theories or methodological refinements or innovations). You should be able to identify which of these aspects will constitute your contribution.

All students find it extremely difficult to determine a methodological plan at a stage when they are still quite uncertain about what they really want to do. The reviewers will not expect the methodology to be carved in stone, but they will expect to be reassured that you are capable of identifying methods described that will meet stated objectives, that your plan of work provides a safety net of work likely to achieve a successful outcome, and that you are not attempting to achieve too much in the time available.

Delimitations and limitations

Delimitations are the boundaries – inclusions and exclusions – which limit the scope of the research (Cresswell, 1994), and these should be established at this stage. They demonstrate to the reviewers the boundaries of the research in control of the researcher or determined by the research problem. This ensures that the reviewers do return the proposal with questions such as, 'Why are you not focusing on...?' Limitations are any potential weaknesses of the research and how these might influence its outcome. You should then indicate how you might compensate for them or overcome them. Far from weakening the study, it demonstrates that you are able to think ahead and pre-empt problems or difficulties.

Ethical considerations

In the health and social care field, ethical issues are particularly important (see Chapter 5). You will be expected to identify all relevant ethical issues, including access to participants, and explain how you intend to deal with these.

Two proposals for submission to research degrees committees

The following are not meant to be templates, but examples of proposals from students working in different disciplines, using different methodologies, and registering at different higher education institutions. They show how two students composed their research proposals, one in the field of biomedical research, the other in the field of medical sociology; one quantitative, one qualitative.

Both proposals included expected starting and completion dates, mode of study (full-time or part-time), details of the background and academic qualifications of the student and academic references (appended); details of research supervisors and advisers with curricula vitae (appended) and supervision experience; programme of related studies including research training, regular seminar programmes, any special courses to be taken and conferences to be attended; collaborating institutions (including NHS and social services or voluntary organisations whose cooperation is essential, in which case letters of consent must be appended); funding sources; special/specialist resources and facilities; detailed time plan for the whole period of study (normally presented in table form); references (note: references in these examples are not contained within the reference list at the end of this chapter).

Example 1: A social science proposal from Bettina Becker (her real name)

Bettina grew up in East Germany and took a degree in sociology in Berlin after unification. German degrees take longer than those in the UK and attain a higher educational level. Although she did not have a professional qualification, she applied for an internally funded PhD studentship in a health studies department of a college of higher education to study the experiences of pain in older people. This expanded on the PhD work of her supervisor, although Bettina was free to decide on the direction of her study. Before enrolment, academic references were taken up and she provided a transcript of her degree for authentication. Her oral and written English were excellent (foreign students are normally expected to take an examination to demonstrate that their English reaches a specified level). She was selected on the basis of her interest in the topic, natural curiosity and commitment to research, knowledge of ethical issues and empathetic interpersonal skills.

Bettina's proposal was developed, after starting her studentship, for submission to an interdisciplinary college research degrees committee. On acceptance, it was forwarded for approval to another interdisciplinary research degrees committee under the auspices of the awarding university. This whole process took about six months, during which time she gained approval from the local research ethics committee, undertook and wrote up a detailed literature review, set about making contacts with NHS gatekeepers, and conducted a pilot study with a volunteer gained through personal contact.

Title of proposed investigation

A biographical perspective on the experience of chronic pain in later life.

Aim of investigation

To investigate how the biography of the individual shapes the experience and meaning of chronic pain in later life.

Sub-aims

(1) To explore and analyse the experience of pain in later life from the perspective of the sufferer (MPhil stage).

Transfer to PhD:

(2) To integrate pain stories and life stories in the analysis of the experience of chronic pain.
(3) To evaluate the significance of biography for the meaning of chronic pain in later life.

Background and related research

Chronic pain in later life is a prevalent distressing condition which has increasing significance due to the growing numbers of older people. At the same time, research on pain has not focused much on the older age group (Melding, 1992: 2; Closs, 1994). Despite the recognition of psychosocial factors on the experience of pain (Walker *et al.*, 1990; Melzack & Wall, 1991; Roy, 1992), most of the research has been conducted from a biomedical perspective (Bendelow & Williams, 1995). Personal narratives have been increasingly used to study the experience of chronic illness (Williams, 1984; Robinson, 1990; Bury, 1991; Kelly & Field, 1996), the experience of ageing (Coleman, 1986; 1993; Haight, 1988; Gearing & Dant, 1990; Haight & Webster, 1995; Stones *et al.*, 1995; Ruth & Kenyon, 1996; Birren *et al.*, 1996) and have been suggested for use in the study of pain (Bendelow & Williams, 1995).

In the proposed research, I will investigate the experience of chronic pain from the perspective of the individuals who are affected. In the analysis of their narratives, I intend to integrate medical, psychological and social factors that shape the experience of chronic pain (see Ellis & Flaherty, 1992; Bendelow 1993). Looking at how the individuals locate this experience in their lives offers access to the interaction of all these factors as experienced by the individual.

Methodology

Narrative interviewing

I will interview persons over 65 years of age who suffer from chronic pain, with the aim of collecting pain stories, life stories and an evaluation of the interview process. Narrative interviews will be conducted in an open way to give the participants scope to speak about their experience choosing their own frame (Kaufman, 1994; Chase, 1995) The interviews will be tape-recorded.

The first interview will focus on the experience of pain and on the present life situation. This will enable the participants to speak first about their immediate experience. In addition, the use of descriptive words for pain from the McGill Pain Questionnaire (Melzack, 1975) will encourage narratives about bodily experience, which are not easy to describe (Olesen, 1992: 211). The analysis of these data will meet the demands of MPhil (sub-aim 1).

In further interviews I will ask the participants for their life stories. The analysis will then focus on the integration of pain stories and life stories to see how the participants locate the experience of pain in the context of their whole lives (sub-aim 2). I will then evaluate the significance of biography for the meaning of chronic pain in later life (sub-aim 3) for PhD.

Theoretical sampling

Potential participants will be accessed via community nurses, according to their identification of good versus bad coping with chronic pain. This criterion will help to increase possible variations in the experience of pain. About ten participants will be accessed as an initial sample. The analysis of the experience of pain (MPhil stage) shall serve to identify further sampling criteria (e.g. class, gender) which emerge as important to increase the variability of the experience of pain in the sense of theoretical sampling (Strauss & Corbin, 1990).

Data analysis

In the analysis of the transcribed interviews, I will focus on the structure of the narratives, the way individuals give coherence and meaning to their experience (Denzin, 1989a,b; Rosenthal, 1995). Rosenthal (1995) offers a detailed method for the analysis of biographical narratives following their internal structure as constructed by the participants during the interview.

The transcripts will be analysed in a small group with colleagues, to enhance the interpretive process.

Ethical issues

The participation in interviews is voluntary, and consent to participate will be negotiated continuously (see Kayser-Jones & Koenig, 1994). All information will be treated as strictly confidential. The interviews can include the recall of distressing events and upset the participant. Interview training is planned to develop interviewing skills to react appropriately and prevent harm to the participants. I will invite an evaluation of the interview process from the participants in the last interview and in one more interview I intend to conduct six months later. Approval from the ethics committee of two NHS trusts has been obtained to access the individuals via community nurses (see appendix). (Bettina Becker, 1996)

Time plan – includes:

- Research training
- Collaborating institutions
- Supervisors and experience (with an explanation)

The appropriate references were added in a separate section.

Example 2 A biomedical proposal from Maria Jones (pseudonym)

Maria Jones was a demonstrator at a university who later became a lecturer.

Title of proposed investigation

Non-enzymatic glycosylation and free radical metabolism in patients with diabetes mellitus.

Aim of the investigation

The aim of this study is to investigate the effect of non-enzymatic glycosylation on free radical metabolism and its role in the genesis of vascular complications in patients with diabetes mellitus.

Background of the project

Introduction

Diabetes mellitus is a relatively common disease with a prevalence of 1–2% in the UK population. Diabetes is costly, not only to the patient in terms of lifestyle and the anxiety of the complications that develop, but also to the nation in financial terms. Clinically, there are two recognised forms. First, insulin-dependent diabetes mellitus (IDDM) which is due to the failure of the beta cells of the pancreas to produce insulin. Secondly, non-insulin-dependent diabetes mellitus (NIDDM) which is probably due to downregulation of insulin receptors. Irrespective of the type, hyperglycaemia is the cardinal manifestation, and it is believed to be an important factor in the development of the long-term complications that affect the major systems in the body.

Previous research

Free radicals (FRs) have been implicated in the genesis of many degenerative disorders, including diabetes (Florence, 1995).

In IDDM, the complications that patients develop are thought to result from microangiopathies that directly involve the vascular endothelium. In contrast, patients with NIDDM have a high mortality from atherosclerotic macrovascular disease.

Microvascular endothelial cell damage, lipid peroxidation and atheroma development are thought to be mediated by free radicals (Darleyusmar, 1992; Pieper *et al.*, 1995; Volk *et al.*, 1995). It is also well documented that hyperglycaemia causes non-enzymatic glycosylation (NEG) of proteins (Lyons, 1992; Suzuki *et al.*, 1992; Beisswenger *et al.*, 1993).

Plan of investigation

The aim of this study is to investigate the effect of NEG on free radical metabolism and its role in the genesis of vascular complications of diabetes mellitus.

The first phase of the project will be to study, *in vitro*, the effect NEG has on superoxide dismutase (SOD) activity. This will entail: *in vitro* glycosylation of the enzyme by incubation with concentrated glucose solutions; separation of glycosylated and non-glycosylated fractions (using electrophoresis or column chromatography); and determination of enzyme activity (using electrochemical and spectrophotometric techniques). This will then be extended to a number of other enzymes involved in FR metabolism.

The second phase of the project will be the transition from MPhil to PhD, and will investigate NEG and FR metabolism in tissue samples from diabetic patients. In patients with IDDM, the focus will be on nitric oxide (NO) and SOD activity of leucocytes as they may have a role in microvascular endothelial cell injury (Huie & Padmaja, 1993). This will require the construction of a sensor for NO measurements. In NIDDM patients, there will be a particular attention to lipid fraction ratios and lipid peroxidation in relation to macrovascular disease (Arauo *et al.*, 1995). In all cases, attempts will be made to relate findings to the patients' glycaemic control as indicated by glycosylated haemoglobin levels.

In patients with foot ulcers, attempts will be made to collect fluid from wound exudates for the analysis of SOD and nitric oxide activity to assess the role of FR in wound development and healing.

Data from this project will help to extend our understanding of the pathogenesis of vascular diabetic complications and will contribute to the development of new therapeutic interventions.

Note: Both the student and the supervisor are experienced in the handling of human tissue samples.

Also included were (but not given here):

- Ethical considerations
- Time plan
- Research training
- Collaborating institutions
- Supervisors and experience (with an explanation)

The appropriate references were added in a separate section.

Timetable planning

One of the most difficult tasks for students is planning and designing a timetable for the research. Universities increasingly restrict the time allowed for PhD studies and specify the minimum and maximum allocated (for instance, at one university the minimum time for a PhD via transfer from MPhil registration is 36 months full-time and 48 months part-time, while the maximum time is 48 months and 72 months, respectively). Sometimes, if valid reasons exist, you can negotiate the time span or suspend your study for a time during the process, but research committees tend to discourage this, except in exceptional circumstances. Suspension is given for serious personal reasons or unavoidable overload in the workplace.

May (1997) makes suggestions about the management of the timetable including:

- Gaining familiarity with the literature in the chosen area
- Formulating the research questions
- Deciding on the research design
- Gaining access to setting and sample
- Carrying out a pilot study (if this is appropriate; in qualitative enquiry this is unnecessary as the process is developmental)
- Collecting data
- Analysing and interpreting the data (in qualitative research, data collection and analysis often proceed at the same time and interact)
- Reviewing the literature (ongoing throughout the research)
- Drafting the thesis
- Finalising the thesis (this includes getting it into its final form and bound)

Each phase of the study should have its own completion date, though it may be revisited. Obviously many of these steps overlap and might change during the research process as more or less time might be needed for each step. Phillips and Pugh (1994), however, advise that the deadlines be kept so that the study can be completed in time.

Fig. 7.1 gives an example of the type of timetable which is useful to include with your research proposal. It allows for parallel aspects of work.

You can set some of your own deadlines; for instance, you can decide what tasks to carry out or what writing to do within one month or three months. It is also important to build in some time to deal with unexpected circumstances such as an illness, operation or unavoidable professional work deadline. Good time management means setting priorities and completing important tasks while leaving marginal work to the later stages.

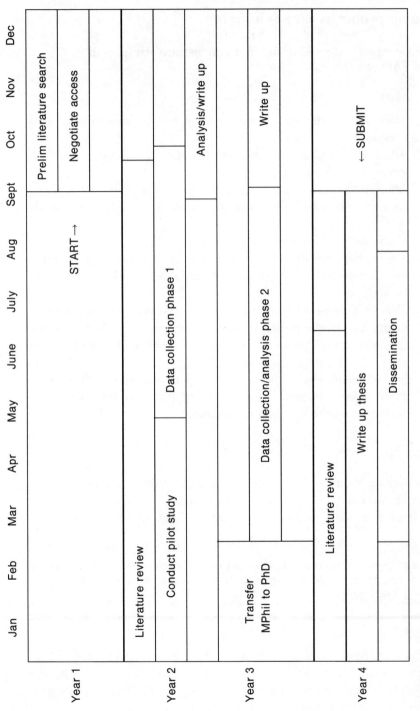

Fig. 7.1 Trajectory.

Some problems and solutions

How can I judge how much I can fit into my period of PhD study?

Solution

- Map out the intended time scale month by month and work backwards from the end.
- Allow several weeks for final proofreading, supervisors' feedback, tidying up and binding.
- Allow a full-time year for final analyses, final literature checking (much of which will be through interlibrary loan) and writing up the thesis.
- Block out your holidays.
- Think about suitable timing of data collection – nobody wishes to be interviewed at Christmas, for instance – think about school holidays, etc.
- Plan each phase of the study in turn, allowing time for reading, theoretical developments, preparation and piloting, data collection (e.g. how many interviews can you reasonably undertake in a day/week?), data analysis, writing up, etc.
- Fit each phase into your overall time plan and see how it works.
- Allow adequate time at the beginning (three to six months) for reading, consultations and preparation.

Comment

Everything about research takes much longer than you originally think it will. Although it is possible to scale down the operation once you have started, it is better to think it through carefully before you start.

I am not certain what I will find in the early qualitative phase of my research, so find it impossible to know how it may develop at a later stage

Solution

Think of the most likely outcome and make your plans around that. It may seem dangerous to pre-empt your findings, but it will give you a security blanket of knowing that what you plan is likely to be do-able. You can always modify or change tack at a later stage.

Comment

Most interesting research involves unexpected and unforeseen developments. The proposal is intended to ensure that you are realistic in your
approach and your expectations. It is not an irreversible commitment.

**I will be working in a number of residential homes to collect my
data. Do I really have to gain permission from all of them
before I start?**

Answer

The research committee which approves your research proposal will
usually wish to be assured that you will have all of the resources you
require for successful completion. They will therefore need to know that
you will be able to gain entry to these types of group home. Letters of
permission from two or three of them and from participants should
reassure the members of the committee.

Comment

It is better to find out at this stage if there are likely to be any difficulties
in gaining access. It is not unusual for managers to be reluctant to
cooperate and they do not have to give reasons for this.

Writing a proposal for an externally funded studentship

Applying for an individual studentship or other source of personal
funding takes time and expert assistance. Do not attempt to do this without recruiting the help of potential supervisors. Successful applicants
have usually been coached and assisted by experts in the field who have
a history of successful applications. It is no good leaving applications
until the last minute. You should normally allow *at least* six months to
plan your application. This allows time for:

- Finding a suitable department and supervisor.
- Holidays and other absence (yours, supervisors', administrative
  assistant's, accountant's, gatekeepers' – it is a good idea to check all
  leave dates at the start).
- Refining the research question and agreeing a suitable methodology.
- Conducting a preliminary literature search and review of previous
  key work.

- Identifying a suitable supervisory team (with external supervisors and advisers where appropriate).
- Obtaining written permission for access to samples.
- Completing the application(s) and gaining written approval from the local research ethics committee(s). Check their dates and deadlines at the start.
- Writing and refining or rewriting the proposal on a photocopied application form.
- Checking the budget.
- Obtaining academic references (you may have to include these with the submission).
- Getting the final application typed up.
- Things to go wrong (something invariably does).
- Gaining the signatures of all concerned.
- Making copies for yourself and your supervisors.
- Posting and delivery (send recorded delivery).

If you allow your supervisor to undertake any of these tasks on your behalf, maintain full responsibility for monitoring their progress. Most supervisors are very busy and even the best are liable to forget. Planning a timetable of events against deadlines is always a good idea.

If the funding agency or council issues guidelines for completion, follow these to the letter. Always type the application (use the computer disk if one is supplied). Never exceed the specified word length. If the guidelines ask for one page of no less than 10-point type size, it means precisely that, and failure to comply will result in swift binning on receipt. Take advice from your supervisor at all stages.

Applicants for NHSE studentships, be they doctors, PAMS, midwives or nurses, compete for a very limited number of awards. The standard is extremely high and it takes intensive preparation. Insider knowledge of the requirements, or previous experience of success on the part of the supervisor is helpful.

Why should I go to all this bother?

With a studentship, you will be cushioned financially for the duration of the studentship. Being able to study full-time enables you to complete much more quickly and enhances your chances of success. These and other less well remunerated studentships are prestigious and lead to excellent employment prospects, in practice, research or teaching, in the long term.

Why will academics want to help me?

Studentships are highly prized by university academics as well as students since they help to influence a department's ratings in the RAE. It helps to keep supervisors' names familiar with the funding agencies and this may help with the success of future funding applications. Also, supervisors like to work with students who have bright ideas and are well motivated.

How should I proceed if no formal guidelines are given?

If you are applying to an agency which does not give formal guidelines, it is a good idea to phone up and ask how long they would like this application to be and what level of detail they would like (e.g. do they need written permissions at this stage?). If in doubt, keep it brief – give the essential details succinctly and logically. The following format may be helpful in ensuring that all relevant information is included.

Format for a research proposal for external funding

This is, of course, not fixed in stone but is intended as a possible starting point. The main difference between this and the academic proposal (above) is that you need to sell yourself and your research and be seen to be addressing important issues for the funding agency. You will also need to provide a budget of likely expenditure.

(1) *Title* (see above)

(2) *Summary.* No more than 200 words, or about a sentence for each of the following points: overview of main aim, rationale (why the study is important), the methodology and why this was chosen, what you hope the outcome will achieve in terms of practical benefit. This is eye-catching and sells your study.

(3) *Aim(s).* State the main aim or purpose clearly, and list any sub-aims or objectives.

(4) *Background.* State why you are personally interested in this investigation. Then give an overview of previous work on the topic, ensuring that you mention all key researchers and theorists in the field (reference these at the end). State how your work relates to previous work. Locke *et al.* (1993) advise not to start

'praising, exhorting and polemicising' (p. 119) in a proposal as this is not its purpose.

(5)   *Benefits.* State how the outcomes of your research are likely to benefit clients or professionals, practice or service (with particular reference to the priorities of the funding agency).

(6)   *Method.* Cover all of the following, using subheadings where appropriate:
   (a)   Design (or type of methodology, indicate if to be conducted in separate phases)
   (b)   Sample (who, where, how many)
   (c)   Ethical issues and how these are to be addressed. Append letters guaranteeing access and letters of approval from relevant ethics committees.
   (d)   Data collection (method and key details)
   (e)   Data analysis (state methods to be used and for what purpose)

(7)   *Dissemination.* State how you will disseminate your findings, e.g. articles in academic and professional journals (state which), conference presentations (state which), study days for professional groups, etc. Allow some time for this in your time plan.

(8)   *Time scale.* Present this in a visual format, using a table or as in Fig 7.1.

(9)   *References.* Numbering system saves space in the text. Cite only key references.

(10) *Budget.* Itemise and justify all likely research expenditure, based on known costs at the time of application, for example:

		Yr1	Yr2	Yr3
(a)	Salary costs (where appropriate with National Insurance superannuation, per annum)	£	£	£
(b)	University fees: three years @ £	£	£	£
(c)	Travel: *n* visits for interviews, average 30 miles return @ 41p per mile	£		
	n visits by rail to supervisors/ advisers @ average £50 return	£	£	£
(d)	Attendance at World Congress (Registration fee, travel, etc.)		£	

		Yr1	Yr2	Yr3
(e)	Photocopying: 500 questionnaires × eight pages @ 2.5p per copy		£	
(f)	Postage: 50 interview letters @ 20p	£		
	500 questionnaires @ 20p		£	
(g)	Administrative help with transcribing: 60 hours @ £6.50 per hour		£	
(h)	Interlibrary loan facilities @ £6 per item	£		
(i)	Computer (give detailed specification and purpose)	£		
(j)	Computer accessories (give detailed specification and purpose)	£		
(j)	Computer disks	£	£	£
(k)	Tape recorder (give detailed specification and use)	£		
(m)	Audiotapes	£		

Give additional justification (no more than a sentence for each) for particular aspects of expenditure where these are not evident above; for example, justify the need for a special software package which is not available within the university. Note:

- Some funders place limits on research costs – do not attempt to exceed these, but do attempt to use all of the money – you will be surprised how expensive doing research actually is.
- Some funders will pay for computers, etc., while others will not – check in their guidelines or, if in doubt, phone them.
- Some funders will pay for conference attendance, while others will not – do check.

Check all budgetary details with the faculty accountant before you submit it, in order to ensure that you have:

- included everything to which you are entitled;
- checked for accuracy;
- covered university on-costs (office and desk space, use of library and computing facilities, stationery, telephone, etc.). These may be included as an add-on percentage or will need to be itemised. If an add-on percentage, check how much the funder allows.

There will normally be a section for your supervisor, supervising department and institution to complete, guaranteeing that you will be given adequate facilities and located in a suitable research culture. Allow time for this to be prepared and included.

Final checks on your application

- Include all necessary elements in your proposal.
- Pay particular attention to the number of hard copies required.
- Ensure all signatures are entered, with full addresses including postal codes, telephone and fax numbers, and e-mail addresses.
- Remember to include copies of all letters of approval.
- Include academic references and supervisors' CVs where required.
- Include the computer disk, if requested.

References

Bond, S. (1996) Preparing a Research Proposal. In *The Research Process in Nursing* (ed. D.F.S. Cormack), pp. 89–101. Blackwell Science, Oxford.

Baker, R. (1971) *The use of operant conditioning to reinstate the speech of schizophrenic patients*. Unpublished PhD thesis, University of Leeds.

Cresswell, J.W. (1994) *Research Design: Qualitative and Quantitative Approaches*. Sage, Thousand Oaks, CA.

Galvin, K.T. (1997) *A nurse-led health education programme for smoking cessation: evaluation using the theory of planned behaviour*. PhD Thesis, University of Manchester.

Locke, L.F., Spirduso, W.W. & Silverman, S.J. (1993) *Proposals That Work: a Guide for Planning Dissertations and Grant Proposals*, 3rd edn. Sage, Newbury Park, CA.

May, D. (1997) Planning time. In *Working for a Doctorate: a Guide for the Humanities and Social Sciences* (eds N. Graves & V. Varma), pp. 59–75. Routledge, London.

Mills, M. (1995) *Narrative identity and dementia: narrative and emotion in older people with dementia*. PhD thesis, University of Southampton.

Phillips, E.M. & Pugh, D.S. (1994) *How to Get a PhD: a Handbook for Students and their Supervisors*, 2nd edn. Open University Press, Buckingham.

Part 2

Progress and Procedures

Chapter 8

Progress, Transfer and Monitoring Processes

Student handbooks

Much of the information contained in this chapter is likely to be found in the student handbook, which you are advised to read periodically. The handbook will generally include the students' responsibilities; the research environment (training programme, supervision from research-active members of staff); the programme of research seminars and facilities; and the pathway through which the students progress to their award. You will be advised of minimum and maximum times for research degrees and the transfer processes from an MPhil to a PhD. The handbook also contains practical requirements for the production of the final thesis including size, colour, margins, spacing and other necessary information. It should also inform you how to obtain pastoral help, should you require it, and advise of grievance and appeals procedures, should this prove necessary. Some colleges and universities have as yet failed to recognise that these formal processes might be necessary for research students. Should your student handbook make no mention of any of these issues, you may wish to pursue the matter through student representation at departmental, faculty or college level (depending on the size of the institution). If you find that research students do not have representation, you may wish to press for its establishment.

Research training

It is essential to ensure that the institution in which you intend to register offers a research training programme which will prepare you to plan and conduct your research and engage in critical debates surrounding the research process. During the last ten years, the ESRC has taken the lead in insisting that all students who hold one of their studentships should devote a large percentage of their time during the first year to research training.

Other agencies have tended to follow the example of the ESRC, though sometimes to a lesser extent, by offering up to a day a week of research training for new postgraduate research students. Most practitioners who have first or Masters degrees in health and social care are unlikely to have sufficient experience of research methods to enable them to plan and execute a full research programme at postgraduate level. It is therefore essential that you check the nature and content of the postgraduate research training programme available to you before you register.

A good general research training programme may include such topics as:

- The philosophy of science and scientific progress.
- Philosophical distinctions between qualitative and quantitative, and inductive and deductive, research methods.
- Critical review of different types of qualitative and quantitative approaches to research.
- The collection, analysis and presentation of qualitative and quantitative data.
- Ethics in health and social care research.
- Guidance on the research process, including administrative procedures. Writing and presentation skills.
- Specialist training programmes designed specifically for health or social care professionals may also include measurement of quality of life and health outcomes; economic evaluation; and social policy issues.

In addition to research training and education, it is important to check that the department in which you are to be located offers a seminar programme in which you may engage in debates about theory and methodology. This should ideally include well-known speakers as well as providing staff and postgraduate students with opportunities to present and discuss their own research.

The Quality Assurance Agency for Higher Education in Britain, in its attempt to promote higher quality in education, has issued a booklet advising universities about their postgraduate research programmes (QAA, 1999). This develops a *Code of Practice for the Assurance of Academic Quality and Standards* which universities are urged to adopt, and on which the members of the agency will focus during quality assurance reviews. This code includes general principles about post-graduate research programmes and other issues. They exhort universities to be accurate in their information and careful in their selection and admission of students, as well as promoting equal opportunities. It would go too far to discuss all the issues in this section, but it is quite clear that they wish students to have access to training in which they can acquire the skills necessary for their research. The booklet also stresses the need of supervisors to have the skills and experience to monitor students' work. Progress of research students must be carefully monitored and communicated. Many other issues are developed in this booklet; you can see that all agencies are concerned to ensure that students have a good research experience at their universities.

Progress and monitoring processes

Figure 8.1 contains an indicative overview of the progress of a typical full-time and part-time student. Of course, there will be variations in progress due to differences in phasing and research approach, unforeseen problems and natural variations in the length of the study. This plan is designed to give some indication of likely or possible progression for guidance purposes only.

Figure 8.1 identifies, in bold, the milestones usually encountered *en route* from enrolment to examination, including annual progress reports, upgrade and approval of external examiners. Although the supervisor has a responsibility to ensure that these are met, even the best supervisors occasionally suffer a memory lapse, and this can lead to last-minute panics for the student. It is advisable to be prepared for these hurdles and, if necessary, remind the supervisor of them. While we recognise that there will be variations in timing, it is useful for you to have some means of pacing yourself. As you progress towards the final examination, you can work backwards from the submission date and allow time for all of the last-minute aspects of preparation of the thesis, including printing and binding.

The annual monitoring process

It is common for universities to have monitoring processes for research students. Apart from appointing supervisors who are your guides and supervise your progress and achievements, research committees or departments generally require yearly progress reports from both

Fig. 8.1 Illustrative guide to the progress of a full-time and part-time MPhil or MPhil/PhD.

Year : Month	Full-time (three years)	Year : Month	Part-time (six years)
Pre-registration period	Topic identified; supervisory team selected; student enrolled in department and university; research proposal written and accepted by Research Degrees Committee	Pre-registration period	Topic identified; supervisory team selected; student enrolled in department and university; research proposal written and accepted by Research Degrees Committee
From date of registration		From date of registration	
0 : 1	Literature review (ongoing)	0 : 2	Literature review (ongoing)
0 : 2	Design data collection tools	0 : 4	Design data collection tools
0 : 3	Establish access	0 : 6	Establish access
0 : 4	Pre-pilot work Start writing up literature review	0 : 8	Pre-pilot work Start writing up literature review
0 : 5	Commence pilot study	0 : 10	**Prepare annual progress report** Commence pilot study
0 : 6		1 : 0	
0 : 7	Analyse pilot study	1 : 2	
0 : 8	Write up pilot study	1 : 4	Analyse pilot study
0 : 9	Plan main study	1 : 6	Write up pilot study
0 : 10	**Prepare annual progress report**	1 : 8	
0 : 11	Up-date literature search	1 : 10	**Prepare annual progress report** Plan main study
1 : 0		2 : 0	
1 : 1	Commence main data collection	2 : 2	Commence main data collection
1 : 2		2 : 4	
1 : 3	Complete write-up to date in preparation for upgrade or first draft of MPhil	2 : 6	Complete write-up to date in preparation for upgrade or first draft of MPhil
1 : 4		2 : 8	
1 : 5	Submit upgrade material* or final draft of MPhil	2 : 10	**Prepare annual progress report**

Contd.

Fig. 8.1 *Contd.*

Year : Month	Full-time (three years)	Year : Month	Part-time (six years)
1 : 6		3 : 0	
1 : 7	**Upgrade from MPhil to PhD or MPhil examination**	3 : 2	
1 : 8	Continue main data collection	3 : 4	Submit upgrade material* or final draft of MPhil
1 : 9		3 : 6	**Upgrade from MPhil to PhD or MPhil examination**
1 : 10	**Prepare annual progress report**	3 : 8	
1 : 11		3 : 10	**Prepare annual progress report**
2 : 0		4 : 0	
2 : 1	Final draft analysis	4 : 2	
2 : 2		4 : 4	Final data analysis
2 : 3		4 : 6	
2 : 4	Commence draft chapters	4 : 8	Commence draft chapters
2 : 5	Select external examiners	4 : 10	**Prepare annual progress report**
2 : 6		5 : 0	
2 : 7	**Approval of external examiners**	5 : 2	Select external examiners
2 : 8	Update literature review	5 : 4	Work on final draft of thesis
2 : 9	Work on final draft of thesis	5 : 6	**Approval of external examiners**
2 : 10		5 : 8	Update literature review
2 : 11	Final proof-reading, printing and binding	5 : 10	Final proof-reading, printing and binding
3 : 0	**Submission of thesis**	6 : 0	**Submission of thesis**
3 : 1		6 : 2	
3 : 2		6 : 4	**Viva**
3 : 3	**Viva**	6 : 6	

*Upgrade material often consists of two chapters of the thesis (literature review and methodology), plus an outline structure for the whole thesis and an abstract of work to date. This may include material which has been submitted or accepted for publication.

supervisors and students. This is why students and supervisors should keep records of the dates and substance of meetings. Record-keeping is particularly important not just for the supervisor but also for yourself for two main reasons: (1) you might wish to refer back to an issue discussed or when challenged; (2) if anything goes wrong there is documented evidence of the process of the research and supervision. It is essential to find out about the procedures at your university at an early stage so that you can plan ahead.

The annual progress report should be taken seriously by all students registered for a research degree. It is their opportunity to specify the progress made to date and to highlight any areas of concern about supervision, lack of progress or reasons for lack of progress. Students are strongly encouraged to be completely honest in completing such forms as they will carry legal weight should any grievance or appeal procedure be considered necessary at a later date. Some research committees are stringent in their scrutiny of these forms, ensuring that the students' report of their progress matches the report of the supervisors. Such committees will invite a more detailed account should there be any conflict of opinion, and may even ask the student to give an oral account. This is good practice, but not all universities take their quality mechanisms so seriously. Where little emphasis appears to be placed on annual progress reports, students are strongly encouraged to write a full account of their own progress and draw to the attention of the appropriate research director or committee any issues of concern.

The transfer from an MPhil to a PhD

This process differs between universities. Most, though not all, higher education institutions have formal procedures for transfer. Sometimes the supervisors and/or the postgraduate tutor of the university make this decision. However, there are several good reasons for formal processes at this critical stage: to review students' work and monitor progress, to satisfy the requirement of the institution and to identify problems at an early stage of the research process. The upgrade occurs up to 18 months after starting the MPhil/PhD (later for part-time students). The supervisors and student together decide on the time of transfer and the readiness of the student who applies to be transferred. The reviewers might be all or some members of the research committee; they might include the supervisor or head of department and often an outsider from another institution with academic and professional expertise in the student's chosen field. Those involved in the transfer process generally do not become external examiners at the final stage so as not to prejudice the examination process.

Before approving the upgrade, the reviewers will ensure that you are likely to achieve a PhD of good standard and quality. The procedure for transfer usually includes a progress report from yourself and a report from the supervisors.

The upgrade report will normally consist of:

- A discussion of the work which has already been carried out.
- A description of how the research question has been defined and followed up.
- Achievement of aim so far.
- Details of the distinct contribution to knowledge the study will make. For students in health and social care, this should demonstrate how the outcome might affect practice or the profession.
- A critical and substantial evaluation of the literature reviewed so far.
- An explanation of how both seminal and recent literature have been used.
- A discussion of the chosen methodology.
- The quality and amount of data collection.
- The data analysis so far.
- The problems encountered and their possible solution.
- A plan for future work including any intended changes.
- Description of the development, modification or generation of theory.

Some institutions require, instead, two full chapters of the thesis (usually an aspect of the literature review and the methodology), together with a written framework which provides a context for the work, details of the method of data analysis with an example to illustrate its application, and an overview of the structure of the thesis.

Many institutions now require students to attend a viva at the transfer stage in which the assessor or assessors ask questions in much the same way as in the final examination. This provides you with an opportunity to discuss your work with independent assessors and also gives you some preparation for your final viva. Although daunting, it is good practice and most students find it extremely helpful.

On the basis of the documentation and the oral assessment (if required), a recommendation is sent to the research degrees committee which will decide if your work is of the required standard to proceed to a PhD. If you are not allowed to transfer, you will be told of the reasons for this and given guidance about what is needed to achieve the required standard. You will also be given a date for the next review for transfer. You need be aware that a successful transfer from MPhil to PhD is no guarantee that the work will eventually lead to the award of a PhD.

Reference

QAA (1999) *Code of Practice for the Assurance of Academic Quality and Standards in Higher Education: Postgraduate Research Programmes.* Quality Assurance Agency for Higher Education, Gloucester

Further reading

Cryer, P. (1996) *The Research Student's Guide to Success.* Open University Press, Buckingham.
Phillips, E.M. (1992) The PhD: assessing quality at different stages of its development. In *Starting Research Supervision and Training* (ed. O. Zuber-Skerrit), pp. 119–135. Tertiary Education Institute, University of Queensland, Brisbane.
Phillips, E.M. & Pugh, D.S. (1994) *How to Get a PhD: a Handbook for Students and their Supervisors*, 2nd edn. Open University Press, Buckingham.

Chapter 9

Avoiding Problems

Problems with supervision

During the course of the research, problems in the academic and personal relationship between yourself and your supervisors may emerge. At the start of a research degree, these problems are more easily resolved. You have, of course, some responsibility to try adapting to a style of tutoring with which you might not be familiar. However, you may have to consider changing supervisors if the first supervisor promotes ideas and suggests approaches which are alien to your thinking. You should first discuss this with the departmental postgraduate tutor or head of department. The research belongs to you, and you have the ultimate responsibility for ensuring its quality and completion. Fortunately, alienation from the supervisor rarely occurs. If it does, you have the opportunity to consult other members of the supervisory team or you might seek help from a senior staff member (such as the departmental research director, or chair of the research degrees committee) in the department, college or university who is likely to be sympathetic and will advise on an appropriate course of action. Some institutions actually have a system of mentoring so that such problems can be dealt with promptly.

If supervisory sessions seem disorganised or problematic in any way at all, you might try to educate your supervisor(s). In most cases, negotiation is possible. After all, professionals are usually good at dealing with different ideas and personalities in the course of their working day and have to bargain and negotiate with those who interact with them professionally, so it might not be difficult to compromise when 'managing' the supervisor.

Problems with supervision might include academic, professional and personal conflicts.

Academic problems

(1) The supervisor is inaccessible or lacks time to see you.
(2) The supervisor gives too little guidance or is uncritical.

(3)   The supervisor is over-directive or gives inappropriate advice.
(4)   The supervisor lacks expertise in the subject matter or methodology.
(5)   The supervisory team members have conflicting ideas about the research.
(6)   The first supervisor leaves the university or is allocated a different role.

Students' most common complaints concern inaccessibility of supervisors. Supervisors are busy people who do not always see the student and supervision as their priority. You can avoid this problem by making an appointment well before the supervisory session or by deciding on a future date at each meeting. Make sure that you inform your supervisors of necessary cancellations. Your supervisors should have your home and work telephone numbers so that they, too, can cancel well before the meeting if they are unavoidably detained or ill. You might negotiate this procedure as part of the contract between yourself and your supervisor.

When students have little guidance, feedback or criticism, they feel uninformed and unsure about their progress or the standard of their work. If the level of help seems inadequate, be honest and discuss this with your supervisor in a friendly manner. Most supervisors are open to helpful suggestions from students. In the end, however, the thesis should be your own independent work. Again, if you are unable to resolve the problem with your supervisor, discuss this with your other supervisors and ultimately the postgraduate tutor or equivalent.

Example

Stan, a speech therapist involved in part-time PhD research, found that his main supervisor was never available because of work commitments, and could see him only rarely. Stan discussed this with another member of the supervisory team who did not wish to discuss his colleague's problems with the student. Eventually Stan had to address the problem by reporting it to the postgraduate tutor of the department who helped him change supervisors.

Students sometimes complain about too much guidance and over-direction. You may feel that the supervisor never allows you to make your own decisions and guides your work in a direction you do not wish to go. Generally, in fact almost always, the supervisor does have the interest of the student at heart and might feel you need strong guidance, particularly in the early stages. Supervisors who are new to the role may do this because they are anxious not to let you down.

A problem sometimes occurs in joint supervision when supervisors have conflicting ideologies and different ideas about the research. Sometimes this is the outcome of misinterpretation. The situation can usually be negotiated. Keep detailed notes of each supervision session. The problem can be avoided if the supervisors are in constant touch with each other and regularly have joint meetings with students.

Quite often supervisors change their roles or move on. They might be promoted to head of department or another position and have little time for the student. They may have a sabbatical or a serious illness. In this case, joint supervision is valuable, because the university can change the position of the supervisory team, allocating the director of studies position to the second supervisor. Usually the first supervisor will stay a member of the supervisory team. Sometimes the first supervisor changes university for career reasons. You might ask the research committee to consider keeping your first supervisor as a member of the supervisory team, and sometimes this request is granted. If not, it is the responsibility of the university to allocate a new and appropriate first supervisor, often a member of the initial supervisory team or a new member of staff. Occasionally, when the first supervisor is one of the few experts in the field of study, the student can transfer to the university to which the supervisor has moved. This is obviously difficult for part-time students who are often tied by personal obligations to a particular location, but can be managed if the student is at a late stage in his or her research and need not see the supervisor very often. Telephone and e-mail tutorials are possible, if not wholly satisfactory.

Professional problems

(1) The first supervisor, although an expert in the field or methodology, lacks understanding of the student's professional interest in the topic.
(2) The supervisor believes that the student has false priorities.
(3) The supervisor is not willing to discuss issues which are linked to the workplace and which have bearing on the research.

Personal problems

(1) The supervisor seems difficult and there is a conflict of personalities.

(2)   The supervisory style does not suit the student.
(3)   The supervisor is unable to develop a relationship with the student.
(4)   The student experiences subtle or open harassment (which may or
        may not be sexual).

Personal problems are the most difficult to resolve in the supervisory
relationship, and they are fortunately rare. They are less significant
when you have several supervisors on whose advice you rely. However,
because the relationship between the supervisor and student becomes so
close – it is usually the most intense academic relationship and often
continues well after the completion of the work – it is important that
the problem is solved at an early stage of the research.

Personal problems may occur when there has been a mismatch
between the supervisor and the student. You might not experience this
problem initially, but it might become obvious after a few months or a
year into the research. In this case, you could try to keep the relationship
on a purely professional basis. If this does not work, you might attempt
to change to another member of the supervisory team so that he or she
becomes the director of studies. Good reasons must be given why you
wish to do so. If there seems to be no solution, this problem has to be
discussed with the departmental postgraduate tutor (or other appropriate individual). The departmental or university research committee
might allocate another first supervisor.

Grievance procedures

Throughout this book, we have encouraged you to think about and
address problems as they arise. In the unlikely event that these cannot
be resolved, you could make use of the formal grievance procedures
available within your institution. Failure to do so could jeopardise the
outcome of your degree.

Problems with the research process

It is difficult, at the beginning of a lengthy research process, to know
which research approaches will work best. Often you need to make
changes as you go along. One of the best ways of ensuring that the work
does not progress too far before the need for such changes are recognised is to ensure that all aspects of the work are properly piloted.

Carrying out a pilot study

Undertaking a pilot project will be useful for the research, although the need for it differs depending on the type of methodology adopted. Locke *et al.* (1993) assure researchers that they can argue more effectively and convincingly when they have tried out aspects of the design with some success and made sure of its viability. The pilot may involve testing an instrument, using a particular sampling frame or carrying out some interviews and observations and so on. Mistakes can be discovered which might prevent the research from being practicable. On the basis of the pilot study, appropriate changes or revisions in the design can be made, such as refining the objectives of the study, decreasing or increasing the sample size or changing the research tool. A pilot study, a practice interview or observation also help focus the study. Some students have had problems because the focus of their research was too broad and all inclusive.

There is no need to carry out a pilot study in a qualitative research project, because the approach is developmental and can encompass early attempts depending on emerging and developing ideas, as long as this is described in the decision trail. It is, however, quite useful to undertake a 'dry run', practising interviewing or carrying out an observation to increase confidence and familiarity with procedures. Just as with the area of study, do not let yourself be pressured by others into adopting a particular research methodology unless you feel competent, confident and interested.

One important suggestion made by Mauch and Birch (1993) is to use available data sets or research tools where possible. For instance, a colleague used the data from the Health and Lifestyle Survey (Blaxter, 1990) to develop a research study on racial issues. Whether you use available data or tools does of course depend on their suitability and appropriateness for your study. Using existing tools not only saves time but can add to the validity and reliability of your findings and ensures that you will be able to compare your findings with those of previous researchers. However, it is always worth piloting any tool to ensure that it really does meet the needs of your study and study population.

Other problems along the way

However well planned and relevant the study, you will meet problems during the research process. It helps to know about some of these so that action can be taken, where possible, to avoid them. In MPhil/PhD research in health and social care, critical issues arise similar to those in other types of research, but it also has its own specific problems. A number of reasons for these problems exist:

- Research is a solitary process, particularly for part-time students.
- It is often interrupted by other activities and life events.
- It needs to be professionally relevant.
- The university procedures are not always clearly documented or organised.
- Research commitments clash with personal commitments.

During the long process of research you might become disillusioned with the topic area, participants may decide to withdraw from the study, your ideas may conflict with those of supervisors and serious life events may occur which interrupt the study and make it seem irrelevant.

The organisation of postgraduate work in the university might also be problematic; for instance, you might not be informed of important changes in procedures or fees, and the relevant committees might be slow in transmitting important information. In some universities, room is severely limited, and postgraduates have little space. Computing facilities also depend on the financial position of the institution. Working from home and balancing demands can be difficult. Some major issues are discussed below.

Emotional demands and difficulties

The path of MPhil and PhD research is not always smooth, and some students experience major emotional difficulties for either personal, academic or professional reasons. Postgraduates go through phases, from high motivation and a keen start through steady stages, to emotional highs and lows. Rossman (1995) calls the process 'an emotional rollercoaster' (p. 40). As long as you are aware of the emotional difficulties, you will eventually be able to solve them.

Feelings of isolation

Carrying out PhD research takes a number of years. Although some postgraduates are members of a work group – such as a group undertaking a biological or chemical project in a lab – most PhD students in the arena of health and social care work on their own on a study specific to their interest and area, even though they might regularly meet other students with whom they can link and discuss the work. The feeling of isolation pervades much of part-time study in particular.

Example

Immy Holloway was enrolled part-time to read for a PhD at King's College, London University. She worked full-time at a university 70 miles away from London and could not attend postgraduate student seminars and lectures because they were incompatible with work time and the responsibility for her family. Even with a supportive husband, she only managed two or three seminars in all the time she was registered. In spite of the help of a good supervisor, she felt completely isolated from other students, not just those in her own discipline.

Many part-time students cannot take part in evening seminars because they live too far away or cannot leave their work for daytime seminars. Initial frustration might be linked to the difficult path of the research proposal which proceeds through a number of internal committees in the faculty and the university before being approved. Although supervisors will have experience of the procedures and views of these committees, expert supervision is no guarantee that the committees will accept the proposal. At this early stage, any setback is disheartening and might dampen the student's enthusiasm, but the study may, in fact, improve through these delays. It will be much more difficult to carry out if the proposal is inadequate or inappropriate.

During the course of the research you might experience a sense of loneliness when you encounter a hurdle in your study. This might take the form of a problem in the data collection or analysis, or when a literature search does not result in useful references. Both of us experienced periods of flagging enthusiasm or felt that we were 'getting stuck', a condition of PhD students mentioned by Phillips and Pugh (1994; p. 77).

Getting bored

Boredom and lack of interest is another problem which sometimes arises during the mid-stage of the PhD, for instance in the second or third year.

It is particularly common for part-time students because of the length of the research process. The source of frustration lies in the repetitive and mechanistic tasks which they occasionally want to shift or avoid altogether. It is difficult to work continuously, and it is a good idea to plan days off from academic study and research. On the other hand, you should keep set deadlines even when supervisors do not pressurise you to do so. Of course, if you carry out research in the biomedical field, deadlines are not just useful markers but are essential for the study and generally determined by the work in hand.

Experience of conflict

The sensitive nature of the chosen research topic may add to the emotional difficulties you experience, especially if you are motivated by reasons close to home.

Example

Julia elected to undertake an MPhil on the impact on women of growing up with a drug-dependent mother. She had, for several years, worked with women who had suffered emotional deprivation or physical abuse during their childhood, some of which appeared to be related to this. But another strong motivation was her personal experience of a drug-dependent mother and the apparent lack of literature on this topic. Her supervisors, aware of the potential problems, tried to dissuade her, but she was quite determined. She advertised for informants and commenced interviews but soon found that the stories of the women she was interviewing brought back painful memories from her own past. Although sympathetic, her supervisor did not seem the right person to talk to about this on a regular basis. Luckily, she found a colleague who was willing to act as a mentor and went to her regularly for debriefing. This enabled her, in turn, to support her informants.

Many researchers in health and social care are women who find great difficulty in juggling time between professional work, research, children and partner. It is often the partner who feels neglected in all of this, and it is not unusual for relationships to suffer as a result. Another complicating factor in this is that higher education can pull women apart from less well educated men, causing resentment. Those who start out with supportive partners may be well advised to sit down with them at the outset and work out how to manage their priorities. No research is worth losing a valuable relationship. Many relationships which fail during the period of study were probably doomed anyway. Nevertheless, the process of breaking up is traumatic and emotionally draining. Supervisors may or may not be sympathetic; some will have seen it all before. It is a good idea, at an early stage, to find an independent counsellor or mentor outside the supervisory team and preferably away from the work environment. All universities have student advice centres or chaplaincies to whom research students can turn for advice and support and who will be very familiar with just these types of problem. Those who do encounter such problems will be well advised to suspend their academic registration as soon as possible in order to sort them out. This will ensure that time does not slip by and deadlines for submission don't become impossible to meet. Degrees committees are normally very sympathetic to these problems, if informed early on.

Writer's block

Occasionally you may experience difficulties in writing chapters or even sections of your research. Indeed, most PhD and MPhil students have writer's block at some stage during the research process. It is a serious obstacle to the completion of the thesis. Initially you have to identify the problem which prevents you from putting pen to paper. Reasons may be:

(1)   Too little confidence and too much anxiety
(2)   The task seems insurmountable
(3)   Lack of organisation
(4)   Too much material
(5)   Too many other demands on your time

(1)   When students are anxious and lack confidence they often procrastinate. The solution is to be rational and realistic. Hall (1994) suggests that students write out a list of tasks and set up a realistic timetable in which these tasks could be completed. The tasks could then be carried out one by one and some of the problems solved. Hall adds that this should be done within a realistic time span so that the student is relaxed and not overly tired. Students should focus on what they *can* do, and this reminder might restore confidence.

(2) When the tasks seem insurmountable because of their size and degree of difficulty, they might be broken down into sections. For instance, it is easier writing a few pages than facing a whole chapter. Different parts can then be integrated at a later stage. Taking small steps helps break down task and time. Sometimes routine work such as collecting and summarising references or transcribing interviews can be useful. Most supervisors and guide books advise that beginning writers do not attempt to write a perfect chapter or document but just start writing (Watson, 1987). Writing is a continuous process and the thesis will be revised and redrafted many times.

(3) If you lack the skill to organise and manage material, you may lose confidence and experience writer's block. The existing material, however, can be reorganised according to a theme. This could be done on the computer so that sections can be shifted and changed at a later stage. Most students have a card system or a field diary in which they note important issues. Sometimes cards contain themes or topic areas with comments. Disorganised notes can be transferred to cards and reorganised. Sometimes students use flowcharts for organising ideas.

(4) 'Drowning in data' is a common phenomenon happening to all researchers, particularly PhD students. You have to differentiate between important and marginal issues and return to the aim of the study to give you focus.

It is daunting when you read too much and end up with overwhelming amounts of material. Hall (1994) maintains that too much reading is an avoidance tactic, particularly when this happens towards the end of the research. To overcome this problem you might stop reading shortly before completing the study.

From the very beginning of the research process, you should not read everything on the topic under study but discriminate and prioritise.

(5) All students, particularly part-timers, have conflicting demands on their time. Friends and family can take up so much time that you feel pressurised and stop working. There is only one remedy, and that means being ruthless, turning down some invitations and

festivities and alerting all friends to be aware that there will be
time for leisure activities as soon as the research is completed.

Example

Joyce was asked, in the first months of her research, to write up her
literature review. By this time, she had read volumes on different
aspects of the topic and found it difficult to know where to start.
She delayed until the deadline was fast approaching. Finally, she
admitted that she was having serious problems with writer's block.
In discussion with her supervisor, she agreed to start by writing up
her own reasons for wishing to undertake the research. This was
actually too long to include in the final thesis, but it did get her
started. Next, she discussed the main issues she had identified in
her literature review and wrote these down as main headings.
Tackling one at a time did not seem so overwhelming. Once she
started, it was difficult to stop and she covered far too much.
Nevertheless, all of this information widened her knowledge base
and helped her to be more selective in preparing the final draft for
her upgrade from an MPhil to a PhD. She later admitted that the
main reason for her writer's block was fear of exposing herself to
criticism from more knowledgeable academics.

Duplication of research by others

You will rarely be the only person in the world interested in the specific
topic, especially if it happens to be on a significant, current and relevant
area in health and social care. This is one of the reasons for staying
abreast with the literature in the field. However, unless you are a scientist
who is on the edge of a major discovery in drug research or has found a
revolutionary treatment that changes clients' lives completely, you need
not feel too worried. Only few researchers have similar aims within the
same topic area, within the same time frame, and with similar participants in the same location. One of the reasons for updating the literature is to find similar studies and use some of their results as additional
data and as a confirmation – or indeed refutation – of the study. Of
course all the major work to date in the field which you have used, must
be acknowledged.

Example

Helen, a part-time MPhil/PhD student, wanted to write an historical analysis of care in the community during the sixteenth and seventeenth centuries. After three years, at the stage of transfer, she discovered from her external assessor that someone had been commissioned to write a book on this very topic and had been given privileged access to scarce archival information. It was too late to change topic and the result was something of a race for Helen to complete her thesis before the book was published. In the event, the book was published first, allowing just sufficient time for her to review its contents in her thesis, relating it to her own work. Helen's PhD examiner was impressed with her critical treatment of the available work and sympathetic to the dilemma posed by the impending book. She passed without need for revision.

There are also risks of your own research being used by others, especially when you do not publish anything until the completion of the thesis.

Example

Chris was in the middle of his research and had discussed many of the important issues with his supervisors. The research was proceeding very well, and some important data seemed to emerge. However, when discussing his research, Chris found out by chance that one of his supervisors had discussed details of his ideas with another researcher. Chris had to stop working on his PhD to be able to publish his findings to prevent the loss of some of his best ideas.

Misconduct

Much advice given to researchers centres on the issues of misconduct. This can take various forms, some of which – though by no means all – are discussed below. Not all forms of misconduct are equally serious but they all involve unethical behaviour. The following include some of these:

- Plagiarism
- Falsely attributing authorship
- Falsifying or fabricating data

The most obvious form of misconduct is plagiarism, which involves claiming authorship when the work has been carried out or written by others. This includes copying sections of text or using other scholars' data without attributing them to their original sources or authors. In particular, anything quoted verbatim must be accompanied by a reference to the author which includes a page number. Plagiarism may go further than simple copying to involve presenting other researchers' or writers' ideas as one's own. Whether accidental or deliberate, this is ethically unacceptable and, if found out, would lead to instant failure or removal of the award.

Some researchers fabricate or falsify their data. The most spectacular example is probably that of the famous psychologist Cyril Burt. Years after his death, other researchers reanalysing his data from twin studies of intelligence (which contributed substantially to the nature–nurture debate) claimed to have discovered that he fabricated some of his data (though this is still in dispute). It may be very tempting to alter such easily falsifiable aspects of the research as the response rate or inter-rater agreement to improve validity or reliability; or ignore categories of response which do not fit the emergent theory. However, honesty is the best policy since the researcher who is found out risks losing all.

Most MPhil/PhD candidates do not deliberately act unethically or fraudulently. It is important, however, to be aware of these issues, so that mistakes can be avoided.

References

Blaxter, M. (1990) *Health and Lifestyles*. Routledge, London.
Hall, C. (1994) *Getting Down to Writing: a Student's Guide to Overcoming Writer's Block*. Peter Francis Publications, Dereham.
Locke, L.F., Spirduso, W.W. & Silverman, S.J. (1993) *Proposals That Work: a Guide for Planning Dissertations and Grant Proposals*, 3rd edn. Sage, Newbury Park, CA.
Mauch, J. & Birch, J. (1993) *Guide to the Successful Thesis and Dissertation*, 3rd edn. Marcel Dekker, New York.

Phillips, E.M. & Pugh, D.S. (1994) *How to Get a PhD: a Handbook for Students and their Supervisors*, 2nd edn. Open University Press, Buckingham.

Rossman, M.H. (1995) *Negotiating Graduate School: a Guide for Graduate Students*. Sage, Thousand Oaks.

Watson, G. (1987) *Writing a Thesis: a Guide to Long Essays and Dissertations*. Longman, London.

Further reading

Cryer, P. (1997) *Handling Common Dilemmas in Supervision.* Society for Research into Higher Education and the *Times Higher Education Supplement*, London.

Chapter 10

Writing Up

Writing should start early on and continue throughout the whole research process. This helps, more than anything else, to reduce the problem of writer's block (see Chapter 9). Although some students leave the writing-up stage until the research is completed, this is a high-risk strategy in terms of successful completion. Wolcott (1990) directs researchers towards planning the thesis from the very first stages of the research. Even though the final structure and approach may have changed dramatically, this initial plan provides a safety net of achievable targets likely to lead to a successful outcome. We would therefore advise you to start writing as soon as possible. It makes the completion of the thesis seem far less daunting. Furthermore, when ideas first develop they need to be recorded or else they are easily forgotten. Even if these early thoughts are not fully formed, they are then available to be developed or redrafted at a later stage. Likewise, early readings, if not recorded, may be difficult, if not impossible, to locate later on. You are left with the uncomfortable knowledge that you read something, somewhere, by someone, which was really relevant and important but which you are now unable to trace. It is extremely difficult to predict, in the early stages of the research process, what will become more or less important as the work proceeds.

Early draft chapters

The background, in terms of what led you to be interested in the study and why it is important to practice, is a good place to start and can be written immediately and from the heart. Even if you later shift the emphasis of the study and need to rewrite it, it is good to have this reminder of where and why you started. It will also help you to establish the rationale for the study, its empirical framework and context before formulating the research design and starting data collection.

The literature review may start out in note form, but it is a good idea to start writing it in essay format from an early stage as this helps to clarify conceptual issues, develop and rehearse theoretical and methodological justifications, and refine the skills of academic writing. Even though you may eventually need to rewrite or exclude much of this early work, you will find it a useful learning exercise and, later on when you come to put together the final thesis, it will come as a relief to find much of this already written.

Many researchers are encouraged to write up their introductory sections for publication as a position or review paper. If you don't feel sufficiently confident to write for an academic journal, why not submit a short paper to a professional journal? The editors are usually delighted to receive this type of work and, unlike academic journals, will even pay you a small fee. It is an excellent way of letting other people know what you are doing. If this is your first attempt, seeing your name in print is most motivating. You may even find, like Jan Walker, that other professionals still write to you years later to let you know of their experiences or find out what you are doing now.

Much of the method section can be written up at a relatively early stage (following the preliminary literature review and acceptance of the research proposal). This includes the justification for the choice of methodology and description of the method, as well as the method of sampling and data analysis. If this is not clear in your mind from the very beginning, mistakes will be made which cannot be rectified at a later date.

Example

Andrew decided to use a grounded theory approach in his MPhil study. While he knew much about qualitative research, he was not fully aware of the importance of theoretical sampling and the interaction of data collection and analysis in this approach. He collected all the data from a predetermined sample and then started analysis, rather than collecting and analysing data as a parallel process so that he could follow up ideas from his emerging theories. His supervisor only found this out after he claimed that he had finished his data collection.

The full method section, including the decision trail, should be completed after the data collection and analysis have been completed. For example, while ethical and access issues may be written up at a very early stage, the ethical and access problems actually experienced, and how these were addressed, will be written in later.

The writing-up process

It is often said that writing is a lonely task, associated with feelings of isolation. However, the word processor has transformed and speeded up the process by making it simple to change words or phrases and move sections around. This should make it so much easier, metaphorically speaking, to commit pen to paper, especially for those already familiar with the keyboard. Both of us learned to enjoy the whole process while writing our theses and subsequent publications – hence this book! But it did not come easily to start with, nor is it always easy now. We often have to put work aside in desperation, returning several days or weeks later when a new idea or slight shift in emphasis has solved the problem and the words flow again. Sometimes a low point in the biorhythmic cycle of intellectual or physical energy completely inhibits writing. Best to leave it, do something else, or take a break. The energy and ideas usually return in due course.

One of the most frustrating things for us and for all part-time professional students is to have to fit reading and writing in around other commitments, rather than being able to concentrate while the ideas are flowing. It is essential to set regular time aside for research in one's busy work schedule. But you may find it best to leave the actual use of this time flexible and allow yourself to 'go with the flow'. Some days are best spent writing sections which require little imagination, such as the method chapter, while others are good for developing and setting out new theoretical ideas. Writing does not necessarily mean starting with the first chapter or working one's way through the thesis systematically and sequentially. Often you perform better when you really wish to work on a development, a problem, something of interest, or when you are passionately involved in an area of data analysis.

The working environment is really important for those involved in writing. Working at home may free you from the interruptions of working alongside others, but brings its own distractions. It also results in the most awful clutter that can annoy the rest of the family. Jan Walker's house was burgled just as she had finished her thesis, and her husband still remembers the embarrassment of explaining to the police that the house had not been trashed by the intruders, but was usually like that. One of the disadvantages of working at home is that work can become intrusive or inescapable. This can lead to feelings of entrapment and even depression. When one of Jan's students experienced such a crisis, she found refuge in the local hospital library (even though she was not a member of staff). This proved to be an oasis of peace and quiet where she was allowed to plug in her laptop computer (such equipment may need to be checked by the hospital electrician) and took regular breaks in the visitors' canteen. One of the dangers of using a word processor is that it is easy to become glued to the screen for hours on end. Do remember to take regular breaks, or it can cause serious headaches, neck problems or loss of energy which can lead to long-term damage to health. Structure your days and weeks with regular breaks for refreshment and exercise. Regular exercise is a wonderful way of promoting physical and intellectual energy.

Although supervisors are expected to read and comment on draft sections of the thesis, they can only discuss, evaluate and guide the study but not write it. The ultimate task of writing is yours alone. Delamont *et al.* (1997) discuss the role of the supervisor in the writing-up process: some interfere too much, others hesitate to give advice. The best supervisor is perhaps one who advises students on writing and rewriting without suggesting too much detail. But all supervisors are different. Some focus on detail, taking their red pen to every error of spelling, grammar, punctuation and presentation. Others are ideas people who comment on lines of argument and logic. The lucky student has one of each! Choose those ideas from your supervisor which you know will enhance your study. But it is your work, so don't be afraid to argue if you feel you can justify an alternative case.

The structure of the thesis

Each thesis will look different and there is no definitive template for how to structure the main content of the study. However, there are some conventions which are helpful. The following guidelines are intended to be broadly interpreted.

The initial section contains the title page, the abstract, acknowledgements and the table of contents, in that order.

Title

As considered in relation to the research proposal, the title should clearly reflect the aim and focus of the research, and may also reflect the methodology used, where this is an important feature. It should be brief and clear and need not include unnecessary terms such as: *A study of . . . An analysis of . . .* as this is inherent and implicit in any research report. Cresswell (1994) suggests that 12 words suffice for a clear descriptive title, though up to 15 may be appropriate in the case of complex studies. Remember, the title is the first information available to other researchers who are conducting their own literature searches, so should convey all essential detail.

Abstract

The abstract of a thesis is a brief summary of the study in around 300 words. It is a most important aspect of the thesis since it appears in the Index to Theses which allows other researchers to retrieve the essential details of your work. It always includes the aim, purpose and rationale for the study, the methods used, including brief details of the sample, the main findings, conclusion and implications. If it helps, put these in as section headings to start with and then take them out once you have included the necessary detail.

Locke *et al.* (1998) claim that the abstract is an extension of the title. There is no need for a long introduction to the topic in the abstract. Avoid vague statements such as 'the findings were discussed' – always give explicit details. References, tables and statistical information are not given.

Example of abstract (from a completed and successful thesis)

This study investigates the impact of a health education pro-gramme on the beliefs and behaviour of a group of patients who smoke and suffer from peripheral vascular disease. The aim of this experimental study was to evaluate whether a nurse-led health education programme had any impact on intentions to smoke, attitudes, behaviour, nicotine dependence and withdrawal. The influence of recent stressful life events and health locus of control on smoking behaviour was also assessed.

A three-group pre-test/post-test control group design was used. Forty-one subjects were randomised to three groups: group 1 – health education with nicotine gum; group 2 – health education; group 3 – usual care (control).

Contd.

Data collection was informed by a number of theoretical sources. Intentions, attitudes and beliefs were measured according to the *theory of planned behaviour*. Smoking behaviour was measured by self-report, end-expired carbon monoxide and urinary cotinine. Nicotine dependence and withdrawal were measured using a nicotine dependence scale and a nicotine withdrawal scale. Stressful life events were measured by a life events inventory and health locus of control was measured using multidimensional health locus of control scales.

At the pre-test (interview 1), baseline data were collected using structured interviews and physiological markers for smoking. The experimental intervention (a four-week health education programme) was introduced to groups 1 and 2. During the programme, data were collected from all three groups, related to smoking behaviour, nicotine dependence and withdrawal and the stressful events both at week two and week three. At the post-test (interview 2), the baseline measures were repeated. All subjects were followed up three months later. Data analysis used a range of non-parametric and multiple-regression procedures.

The theory of planned behaviour provides a valuable conceptual framework for examining the impact of health education. Some evidence is provided to support the assumption that perceived control over stopping smoking is an important factor in smoking cessation. Although the hypotheses concerning the effects of the health education programme cannot be fully accepted, the findings demonstrate that the programme did have some impact on intentions, attitudes and behaviour. It is not possible to draw any conclusions about the role of nicotine gum in this programme. The study highlights the importance of the nurses' role in helping people form intentions to stop smoking and raises issues about the nature of health education evaluation. (Galvin, 1997)

Acknowledgements

In most theses, those individuals who helped with the study are acknowledged. This might include the funding agency, supervisors and advisers as well as those who gave statistical support. Do remember to write down their names during the course of the study or you may find yourself in the embarrassing position of having forgotten important names or titles. Some students mention supportive parents, partners, spouses or children.

Table of contents

Write this last – after the final draft has been approved. This saves many mistakes from forgetting to alter page numbers from previous drafts. The table of contents contains a list of the major headings and subheadings. Depending on your judgement, it may be long or short. If subheadings are included, it is easier for readers of the study to find the specific sections. Many follow the convention of numbering chapters, sections and subsections; e.g. Chapter 1 progresses through sections 1.1, 1.2, etc. with subsections 1.1.1, 1.1.2, etc. This can help readers to orient themselves and locate material, but do be careful that it does not become too cumbersome. Only insert such a numbering system in the final draft. Inclusion in the early stages can disrupt the writing style and result in the frequent need to change it. Overzealous numbering may, however, disrupt the storyline in a qualitative study.

Tables and figures are included separately at the end of the table of contents. Rather than numbering (and then renumbering on revision) these through the thesis, it is saves a lot of time to use a convention of numbering them within each chapter. Thus the second table which appears in Chapter 3 is Table 3.2.

Appendices appear at the end of the thesis, after the reference section, and are usually numbered separately, often using roman numerals. A separate contents to appendices at the beginning of these may be helpful.

A useful tip is to use tinted paper, such as buff, to distinguish the appendices from the rest of the thesis, although not all institutions allow this. This enables the reader to locate the reference section (the last of the white pages) and the appendices much more quickly and easily.

Glossary/definitions

It is helpful to the reader who does not share the same background as the candidate to be able to refer to a separate section in which terms, expressions and abbreviations are defined. These may be inserted before or after the body of the thesis.

The body of the thesis

This normally contains

Introduction

- The aim of the research
- The problem statement, background and rationale for under-taking the study
- Critical review of relevant literature, divided into appropriate sub-sections
- Summary and statement of specific research questions, objectives, hypotheses

Method

- Rationale for choice of methodology
- Study design
- Sample, including method of sampling
- Instruments/measurements (where appropriate)
- Ethical considerations (these inform the process of data collection)
- Method of data collection
- Method of data analysis
- Consideration of validity and reliability, limitations and delimitations (Rigour, trustworthiness and authenticity will also have to be discussed in qualitative research)

Findings or results (these may appear as a series of chapters)

Discussion (in qualitative studies findings and discussion are often integrated)

Conclusions
- What has been learnt?
- Implications for practice

Each of the above sections is discussed below in more detail.

Introduction

The introduction to the thesis generally contains a number of sections presented separately or, more often, integrated.

- The aim of the research
- The problem statement and the context
- The background or rationale for the research
- The boundaries of the research
- The importance of the study for clinical practice/clients/the profession

The aim

It is a good idea to start with a broad statement of the research aim to help orientate the reader. More specific aims, objectives or hypotheses are given after the literature review, once the gaps in knowledge have been established. The aim of the study is what you wish to find out through doing the research.

Examples

The aim of this research was to explore (examine, compare, test) ... in order to ...

The ultimate goal need not be stated, but readers might find it useful to see an immediate purpose to the study in terms of practice-related or professional outcomes. The potential outcome of the research can be explained during the introduction.

The problem statement and background

The problem statement relates to the issue or problem addressed in the research and provides the reader with a contextual overview and justification. The context may contain:

(1) *Professional background.* A personal introduction of up to a page in length is an excellent introduction to a professional MPhil or PhD. It greatly helps the reader to know how experiences have come to shape your beliefs and intentions, and the context in which you intend to apply the research. If you have developed your own research ideas from an aspect of practice, it is a good idea to write this section in the first person (see Webb, 1992; Winkler & McCuen, 1994).

(2)   *Empirical framework*. This may include epidemiological or survey evidence to support the scale of a health or social problem, or a piece or research which has promoted the need for further investigation of the issue in question.

(3)   *Social and historical background*. The effects of social or policy changes, events and processes which have an impact on the study could be discussed.

(4)   *Theoretical framework*. Initial philosophical and theoretical assumptions and ideas which are likely to be challenged or developed during the course of the study.

Critical review of relevant literature

This part of the introductory section is where you present and evaluate current and seminal literature on or of direct relevance to the research topic. This provides a framework and justification for the research. Rudestam and Newton (1992) suggest the use of subheadings which are sufficiently explicit to indicate the content of each section to the reader. This generates a clear structure for the review and shows the reader that it has been carried out systematically. You can link your own work to the existing literature and demonstrate how past and current research has neglected the particular problem (situation, event, location or sample) under study. Through describing the deficiencies and limitations of the existing literature, you are able to point to the gap in knowledge (in terms of theory, methodological approaches or information) which you wish to close. Thus the basis for the MPhil or the PhD is made explicit for the reader.

Summary and statement of objectives

Finish with a review of the main findings of the literature review and a statement of the objectives of the study or the reasons for the next chapter if, for example, this will explore methodological consideration.

Method

The main purpose of this chapter is to enable replication by other researchers or to assist them to follow the decision trail. This section must therefore be comprehensive, clear and concise. It is normally presented under subheadings which will be familiar to other researchers and ensure that no relevant information is excluded.

Design

The design is the overall plan of the research, details of the chosen methodology, the approach and the principles behind the research. The design of the research must be closely linked to its aim and research question and explicitly justified. It is important to ensure that the research question determines the methodology, not vice versa. Avoid writing an essay about the methodology, but do ensure that you reference your sources and say how existing approaches were applied or modified.

Where you may have spent some time considering alternative methodological approaches and wish to expound these considerations in your thesis, it may be helpful to insert an additional chapter prior to the method chapter entitled 'Methodological considerations'.

Sample

The sampling process (random, purposive, etc.) must be clearly stated and justified in accordance with the chosen methodology and study design. The size and type of sample must be adequate to achieve the aim of the research and support the conclusions. The sample may consist of events, situations, materials, documents or people. This section includes why and how the sampling units were chosen. You should describe where you located the sample and how you obtained access to it. Inclusion and exclusion criteria are stated. This is also the place where a discussion takes place about the problems encountered while sampling and how they were solved.

Details of sample size, demographic details (such as gender, age, social background) and other relevant detail must be included to enable comparison with previous or future research. Quantitative studies will normally include age range, mean and standard deviation, while qualitative studies should provide some indication of age range.

It is worth noting that the British Psychological Society has discouraged the use of the term 'subject' in favour of participant or respondent. Qualitative researchers never use 'subject' (see Morse, 1991). The term now has politically incorrect connotations of experimental manipulation and appears to have no place in research in the sphere of health and social care.

Instruments/measurements

All measurement instruments, including questionnaires, must be clearly identified and, where appropriate, referenced. All innovations or modifications must be clearly explained and examples given. Questionnaires, interview schedules or interview guides are referred to and included in an appendix. In qualitative research, the researcher is the tool of data collection and this section, suitably retitled, may be an appropriate place to describe and justify the interview technique used.

Ethical issues

The section on ethical issues is located where most appropriate. Since it informs the process of data collection, it seems logical that it should precede it. It should not be a general discussion of ethics but an explanation of how you have considered these issues in relation to the research, together with any specific problems and concerns which arose, and how you dealt with them. Where the study involves a sensitive topic, it might be included as a separate chapter, or discussed in a chapter entitled 'Methodological considerations' which could precede the method chapter. Applications and responses from ethics committees should be placed in an appendix and referred to here.

Data collection

The process of data collection is described in detail, together with the data sources and recording procedures. This includes all actions which you carried out to enhance cooperation and response rates. Letters to gatekeepers and participants should be referred to here and included in an appendix. Problems encountered and how these were dealt with should be given. This is also a suitable place to report the response rate.

Data analysis

You need to describe the way in which you analysed the data, including the organisation and management of the data and any instruments used (including computer software). In qualitative research, data collection and analysis often interact, and this has to be made explicit, step by step. In quantitative research, the statistical techniques used must be described and justified.

Validity and reliability

Most theses have a section on validity and reliability (or their equivalent in qualitative research). The reliability and validity of the research instruments can also be reviewed in the 'instruments/measurements' section.

Delimitations of the research

It is a good idea at this point to state the delimitations of the research, its boundaries. This clearly signals your intentions to the reader and ensures that they do not have unrealistic expectations of the results or findings.

Results or findings

In quantitative research, the results consist of a series of factual statements of the outcomes of the analysis, accompanied by statistical information (including the test statistic, degrees of freedom and one- or two-tailed probability level). Rossman (1995) suggests to researchers that the results are reported in 'narrative' format, adding diagrams, graphs or tables as appropriate. At this stage there is no interpretation, evaluation or elaboration (although this may be different in qualitative research where the findings and discussion are often integrated, but do take advice from your supervisor on this). Readers should be able to assess the findings and form their own conclusion from the factual presentation. Some raw data, such as computer printouts which have been tidied up and reduced in size, may be given in an appendix to illustrate the analytical process. Negative results must be reported alongside positive results. The sequence of presentation should follow a logical structure in which related issues are grouped together.

If you are reporting the results of computer analyses, use full variable names. Never expect the reader to remember what Q1 (question 1) referred to, nor expect them to look this up in the appendix. Variables acquire abbreviated names because packages such as the Statistical Package for the Social Sciences (SPSS) cope only with eight digits. These abbreviations have no intrinsic meaning and must be related back to the original questions for the purposes of reporting in text and tables. Ensure that all tables are clearly labelled with legends and titles, so that they stand alone for the reader to browse.

In qualitative research, the findings are normally grouped according to emergent themes or issues, each supported by data such as quotations or fieldnotes from observations and discussed in relation to existing literature.

Discussion

The discussion includes the reflection on the findings and their interpretation. (Findings and discussion are often integrated in qualitative studies where researchers have more flexibility.) Try to follow the same logical sequence of presentation where appropriate – don't jump about. The discussion focuses on the findings directly derived from the data and is not based on speculation or unfounded inferences. Unexpected findings and those that do not support the initial hypothesis need particular attention. During the discussion, the findings are linked to the relevant literature, most notably a comparison with the findings of previous studies and the extent to which gaps in knowledge have now been filled or previous problems can now be explained. Concepts and theoretical perspectives related to or emerging from the research are developed here. It is important not only to discuss the findings one by one, but also to show that the research forms a coherent whole.

The discussion should include a section in which the strengths and weaknesses of the study are considered, including the validity and reliability (or equivalent) of the findings and any limitations of the work. These issues will determine the robustness of the conclusions and implications for practice. It may also be relevant to include a section on personal reflections on the study, identifying how you might improve it if you were to start again (though be careful not to denigrate your achievements).

Conclusion

The conclusion is a summary of what you learnt from and during the research. Locke *et al.* (1998) claim that the conclusion 'is not the output of some mechanical operation' (p. 86) and 'only the researcher can reach a conclusion' (p. 87). Supervisors or readers can only evaluate the study on what they can see, hear or read. In the conclusions you should list the findings and the points that have arisen from them, in logical order. If you have generated new and surprising findings you will be able to highlight these and explain their meaning. It is preferable not to include new references at this stage – such material should have been addressed in the discussion.

The conclusion provides an answer to the research question. It must link directly to the aim of the research, the methods adopted and the results. A common mistake is to go beyond the findings at this stage into the realms of speculation. Occasionally, you might be tempted to report what you wanted to find, rather than what you actually found. This is a recipe for failure at MPhil or PhD. It is better if the conclusion does not contain rigid statements and remains somewhat tentative. Never be tempted to proselytise and avoid the word 'should' (for example, 'on the basis of these findings, physiotherapists should...'). Identify gaps which still emerge from the research, though be careful not to invalidate your own work. On the basis of the conclusion you might make recommendations for further studies.

Implications and recommendations for practice

As the research was concerned primarily with a problem related to health or social care, and was intended to help clients or the profession, there must be implications for practice which are directly based on the conclusions. At this stage, you could explain how the original problem may be solved as an outcome of your research and highlight some of the problems you or others might encounter when attempting to implement some of the recommendations in practice. It is advisable to end on an upbeat note, reflecting on what you have gained in personal terms from this research.

References

This section includes all material cited, from books, articles and other sources. Check carefully to ensure that it provides a perfect match with text references, is complete in terms of detail, and conforms to the referencing system recommended by your faculty or university.

Appendices

These include supplementary material including letters of permission from ethics committees and participants (with names and locality blocked out). A detailed list of participants with their characteristics such as age, gender, location or any relevant factors can be attached, but care must be taken that individuals or places are not identifiable. Tables or diagrams, tests or other examples of research instruments, as well as questionnaires or interview schedules and guides which have a bearing on the thesis, but need not be integrated or interrupt its flow, can also be included in an appendix. It is better if the study does not contain too many lengthy appendices.

We advise that those undertaking qualitative research include one complete interview transcript which illustrates their interview technique. They may use this transcript as an example on which to base a critique of their performance.

Final preparations for submission

Tidying up the thesis after completing the final draft requires time and effort at a point when both are usually in scarce supply. It is useful to engage help with the final proofreading, including checking the references and appendices. Leave writing the abstract and contents sections until last, but remember to check these too, particularly if you need to make any last-minute alterations.

At this stage, you also need to ensure that you have rigorously adhered to all of the guidelines for submission provided by your university.

Judging a good thesis

A good thesis should be a good read. In fact, it should read in the same way as a detective thriller. A problem is identified – it needs a solution; evidence is brought to bear to justify the need for the investigation; the plot thickens – the nature of the problem becomes clearer; an investigation is definitely required; an investigation is proposed, its detail described and carried through – what will it find? – the findings are presented and answers start to unfold; eventually, all is revealed – the problem is solved, or further problems are identified. There is a tidy ending in which the problem has been addressed and the reader feels satisfied that a sound conclusion has been reached.

A good thesis will be written in plain, accessible English which is easy to follow. Irritating typographical errors are kept to a minimum. The line of argument is clear and sustained throughout; the flow of text is maintained and developed so that the reader's attention and interest are maintained until the end.

Anything that distracts the reader or disrupts attention will annoy, draw attention to detail and promote 'nit-picking'. A free-flowing text which sticks to the main thesis allows the writer to get away with many minor irregularities. Indeed, a reader whose attention is firmly gripped often fails to spot even fairly obvious errors. It is sometimes difficult for the student who is so familiar with the work to be aware of disjunctures or omissions in the line of argument, particularly in the introductory sections. Supervisors will help spot these, but invite someone else to read it through as quickly as possible and just place a question mark in the margin every time they feel lost or stuck. Then go back and address these.

Tips to help you avoid unnecessary criticism from the examiner are:

- Make sure you define all terms (in a few words) that might not be understood.
- Avoid unnecessary repetition.
- Be succinct; remove all redundant verbiage on rereading.
- Never offer more than two linked propositions in a sentence. Break up long sentences into smaller sentences.
- Avoid or eliminate redundant or irrelevant information, even if you spent a long time gathering it.
- Link all sections and chapters together with a sentence or short paragraph so that the reader knows what to expect next and why.
- Never expect the reader to remember small but important detail (e.g. the age or occupation of a respondent, or to which variable 'ADAT' was intended to refer).
- Stick to the same logical order of presentation, as far as possible, throughout the introduction, results and discussion.
- Avoid using 'the researcher' or 'the experimenter' to refer to yourself.
- Avoid the use of 'we' as in 'we can see' – the reader is tempted to say, 'speak for yourself'.
- Set out all of your theoretical or methodological assumptions clearly.
- Let your thesis emerge demonstrably from your analysis, rather than your preconceptions.
- Try to write for a sceptical reader who is generally very well informed, but not entirely familiar with specific aspects of practice, theory, methodology or analysis.
- Avoid any temptation to proselytise, even if you feel passionately about an issue.

References

Cresswell, J.W. (1994) *Research Design: Qualitative and Quantitative Approaches*. Sage, Thousand Oaks, CA.

Delamont, S., Atkinson, P. & Parry, O. (1997) *Supervising the PhD: a Guide to Success*. Society for Research into Higher Education & Open University Press, Buckingham.

Locke, L.F., Silverman, S.J. & Spirduso, W.W. (1998) *Reading and Understanding Research*. Sage, Thousand Oaks, CA.

Morse, J.M. (1991) Subjects, respondents, informants and participants. *Qualitative Health Research* 1, 403–406.

Rossman, M.H. (1995) *Negotiating Graduate School: a Guide for Graduate Students*. Sage, Thousand Oaks, CA.

Rudestam, K.C. & Newton, R.R. (1992) *Surviving your Dissertation: a Comprehensive Guide to Content and Process*. Sage, Newbury Park, CA.

Webb, C. (1992) The use of the first person in academic writing: objectivity, language and gatekeeping. *Journal of Advanced Nursing* 17, 747–752.

Winkler, A.C. & McCuen, J.R. (1994) *Writing the Research Paper: A Handbook*. Harcourt Brace, Fort Worth.

Wolcott, H.F. (1990) *Writing up Qualitative Research*. Sage, Newbury Park, CA.

Further reading

Brown, R. (1994) The 'Big Picture' about managing writing. In *Quality in Postgraduate Education* (eds O. Zuber-Skerrit & Y. Ryan), pp. 90–109. Kogan Page, London.

Glatthorn, A.A. (1998) *Writing the Winning Dissertation*. Corwin Press, Thousand Oaks, CA.

Torrance, M., Thomas, G.V. & Robinson, E.J. (1993) Training in thesis writing: an evaluation of three conceptual orientations. *British Journal of Educational Psychology* 63, 170–184.

Chapter 11

The Examination

Submission of the thesis

To obtain the MPhil or PhD, you are responsible for handing in a thesis of appropriate quality and standard and must then present yourself for a viva voce to discuss and defend your research. In most universities, theses may be submitted in a temporary binding for the examination (see the regulations of your university). Generally they are bound by 'perfect binding' where pages are glued together at the spine so that pages cannot be added or removed. Most research offices ask for three copies. Remember to keep one for yourself and a copy for each of your supervisors. If you have any publications to your credit, place a copy of each in a pocket inside the back cover. In its final form, once approved by the examiners, the thesis must be in a permanent hard binding. A minimum of three copies is required, one of which is placed in the university library, one is sent to the British Library and one is returned to you. Most students also supply a final copy as thanks to their main supervisor. Nurses often choose to place a copy in the Steinberg Collection at the Royal College of Nursing so that it is accessible to other nurse researchers.

You have the right to submit the thesis for examination at any time after the obligatory minimum period has elapsed and before the expiry of the registration period. Although most institutions suggest that it is the student's responsibility to decide on the completion and readiness of the thesis (Cryer, 1997), it would be unwise to hand in the work before it has been approved for submission by the supervisory team and the departmental research committee. On the other hand, the ultimate decision rests entirely with you. It is expected that you are fully aware of the requirements and procedures as well as the potential recommendations of the university and the general expectations of examiners for the research award. The procedures will be described in the research students' handbook. The minimum time from submission to viva is usually six weeks, in order to give the examiners adequate time to read and digest the work. In reality, a delay of three months is not unusual, simply in order to find a date agreeable to all concerned.

Choice of examiners

Examiners are generally chosen by the director of studies in consultation with other members of the supervisory team and often the student. The examiner is then contacted, but must be approved and appointed well in advance of submission by an examinations board within the university. The examiners are required to send in a CV, giving evidence of their suitability and experience to act as examiners on the topic. Each university will have its own set of criteria stipulating, for example, the previous examining experience of the external examiner or the examining team. In UK universities, at least one internal examiner (an academic from your own institution) and at least one external examiner (an academic from another university) are involved. This is different in the USA and some other countries, where all examiners might be internal to the university.

The role of the external examiner is to ensure that the thesis, as defended at viva, meets the required standard, as judged against those of other universities (the criteria have already been discussed in Chapter 1). The role of the internal examiner is to ensure that the standards of the awarding university are upheld. Externals are usually experts or specialists in your field of study. You can expect, at the very least, the team of examiners to be knowledgeable about the general topic area and the methodology adopted in the research. External examiners often have more specific knowledge directly related to the students' work, while internal examiners are more concerned with the general area of the work (Elton *et al.*, 1994). It is sometimes difficult to find an internal with in-depth knowledge of your field because the recognised expert was appointed as supervisor. However, internal examiners are selected from those members of university staff who have either specialised, or at least general, knowledge of the subject area and the methodology. They should not have been involved directly in your supervision.

There may be particular problems in identifying suitable external examiners for candidates in the field of health and social care. Firstly, there are likely to be relatively few people who meet the required criteria with respect to qualifications, suitable academic expertise and previous examining experience. In the UK this is due to the fact that research degrees in some fields of health and social care (in nursing, physio-therapy and social work, for instance) are relatively recent. Gaining experience and undertaking a research degree, as well as supervising students through successful completion of MPhils and PhDs, takes a long time for academics and professionals in these areas of study. Secondly, much research in health and social care crosses traditional disciplinary boundaries and may be multi- or interdisciplinary. One of us (Jan Walker) had three external examiners for her PhD because her research involved nursing, health psychology and gerontology. Although a single external examiner could have been appointed from any one of these disciplines, the advantage was that Jan gained recognition within all three disciplines. However, Phillips and Pugh (1994) in their definitive book 'on how to get a PhD' warn that, the more examiners are involved, the more likely a weak thesis is to fail. Jan's examiners each focused on different aspects of the thesis. One was completely satisfied, one made a tentative recommendation for an inclusion in the appendix, while the other required additional theoretical material to be included in the introduction.

Customarily, candidates know the names of their examiners well before the submission of their thesis and arrangement of the viva. Externals often have prior links with the university or the supervisors. The supervisor does sometimes involve the student in the choice of external examiner, and there is nothing wrong or inappropriate in this. After all, MPhil and PhD students are often best placed to know the names of experts in their areas of research, their methodologies and their stance to the topic. We know of cases where the student suggested an examiner because of his or her eminence in the field and expertise in the particular methodology. However, you should not have a personal or prior academic relationship with the external examiner so that fair judgement of the thesis is not jeopardised. It is worth remembering that the standing of the external examiner(s) is sometimes used as an indi-cator of the quality of the MPhil or PhD. Furthermore, if the externals are impressed with the work, they can become useful contacts or collaborators for postdoctoral research, or assist with advising of future employment opportunities.

Most universities demand that the external examiner has substantial experience in examining research degrees (they usually gain their experience as internal examiners). If you are a member of staff, the university generally requires two external examiners. It is advisable to be well aware of the rules and regulations about the examination and the appointment of examiners. The supervisors, who may not always recall every element of the handbook, occasionally make mistakes. These can be avoided if you keep up to date with regulations.

Example

Joan, a university lecturer, had finished and submitted her thesis for examination. The supervisors and departmental research committee were late in submitting the name of one external and one internal examiner to the university research degrees committee. In giving approval, the degrees committee reminded the department of the requirement that staff members should have more than one external examiner. The search for and approval of another member of the examination team delayed the viva considerably. Joan eventually had her viva seven months after submitting the thesis. The fault lay with the supervisory team and the examinations secretary, but Joan could have avoided the problem by reminding her supervisors of the rules and requirements.

Examination criteria

External examiners should judge the MPhil or PhD thesis against established criteria, some of which are generated by the thesis itself (for instance, the conclusions should answer the research question and be based on the use of a suitable research methodology). We have already discussed criteria for judging an MPhil or PhD (Chapter 1), using guidelines published by the HEFCE and organisations such as the British Psychological Society (UCoSDA, 1995). The awarding institution will also have published clear guidelines. You should acquaint yourself with these prior to submission, in order to make sure that you have met the requirements for the award; and reacquaint yourself with them prior to the viva, since they may help to inform you of likely lines of questioning.

The tasks of examiners

The examiners' tasks consist of the following:
(1) They read the work in detail, evaluate it and make notes about it.
(2) They are usually asked to report independently on the quality and
     standard of the research in a letter to the candidate's university

well before the viva (neither the student nor the supervisor normally sees this).

(3) On meeting, immediately prior to the viva, the members of the
examining team agree the main areas of questioning.

(4) They give the candidate an opportunity to discuss these key areas
of the research and justify their work in detail.

(5) In applied research with policy or professional implications, they
ask candidates to demonstrate the implications and usefulness of
their research.

(6) They question the candidate about the relationship of theory to
practice in their professional field.

(7) After the viva they discuss and report jointly on the quality of the
candidate's work.

(8) They immediately inform the candidate of their decision.

(9) They send their joint evaluation to the relevant committee or
secretary of the university in which the candidate is enrolled.

The viva voce

The viva voce, or 'viva', is the oral examination, the critical part of the
examination process for an MPhil or a PhD. The viva normally takes
place at the institution in which the student has been registered, though
occasionally, if there are time constraints, it is held on the external
examiner's premises. You can usually take your own copy of the thesis
to the viva. (If you have found typing, spelling or other errors, you
might bring these on a separate sheet and inform the examiners of
corrections.)

Those present will include the external examiner(s) and the internal
examiner(s). There may be an independent academic member of
university staff in the chair. The first supervisor is often present, subject
to your agreement, but will not normally be involved in examining. You
might consider allowing the presence of the supervisor for several
reasons. First, it is reassuring to see a friendly and supportive person
whom you know well. Second, it allows the supervisor to assist you,
should revisions be required as a result of the viva. Third, through
attendance at the viva, the supervisor can enhance the supervision of
future candidates by listening to a variety of different examinations and
taking note of style and content. Last, but not least, it is a reward for the
supervisor to experience your success when you do well, manage to
defend your thesis and justify results and methods.

The viva normally lasts between one and two hours, though it may be longer depending on the decisions of the examiners. It is a verbal justification of the work and has a number of purposes:

(1) The examiners use it to give you an opportunity to discuss the research findings and methodology.
(2) The examiners can probe your depth of understanding.
(3) You have the opportunity to defend what has been written.
(4) The examiners can ascertain that the thesis is your own work.

You are normally given the opportunity to justify and give reasons for the choice of topic, to explain your aims and place the research in context. This is particularly important in the health and social care field because the research has generally been carried out for its application in practice. You can demonstrate verbally how you arrived at your findings. Through asking questions and probing, examiners make certain that the research is your own and represents individual work.

Although we cannot predict the areas in which the examiners will ask questions, or the direction of the viva, it is likely that some of the following issues will be discussed in relation to the thesis:

- The choice of topic and approach
- The content of the work
- The theoretical issues that emerged
- Methodological questions and problems, including choice and application of research tools
- The findings of the research in relation to its aim
- The interpretation of the data and the findings
- Problematic issues in the research or the thesis
- The contribution that it makes to knowledge in your discipline or field of study
- The relevance and implications for professional practice

Not all of these questions will be addressed in each case. We know of candidates who were not asked anything about methodology, others who did not have to discuss the implications for practice, but you do well to prepare for all eventualities. Just occasionally examiners ask questions not directly connected with the thesis but with the wider field. This happens rarely, but you should be aware of the possibility, so that you can draw on your wide reading in the area of research. For professionals in the field of health and social care who are carrying out applied research, it is important to be aware of all the implications for practice. Examiners might ask about this, and you should be able to demonstrate that your work is not 'blue skies' research but applied to practice and directly useful.

In a good viva, you will be able to clarify certain questions and verbalise implicit ideas, thereby achieving the final aim of the MPhil or PhD. Burnham (1994) stresses that a good viva cannot make up for a flawed and severely limited study. On the other hand, a competent thesis might be seen in a different and negative perspective if you completely lack confidence and do not answer questions appropriately during the viva.

Example

Tony, a social worker and part-time MPhil student, had submitted his thesis and presented himself to his examiners for the viva. Although having some reservation and criticism about his ideas, the examiners were ready to award his MPhil as the study appeared to provide evidence of a reasonable standard of competence. Tony was very nervous during the viva. He seemed inarticulate and unable to defend his work; indeed, he was mute much of the time. The examiners were unable to pass his thesis and decided that more work was needed for the MPhil to be awarded. They specified certain changes and demanded that Tony make his tenets and ideas more explicit.

It is necessary to differentiate between articulateness and verbosity, as well as between appearing calm and being speechless. The best way is to debate the issues on which challenged with confidence, to answer criticism without arrogance, and to make thought explicit. Do pause to gather your thoughts, if that helps. Through the viva you will be able to demonstrate in-depth knowledge of your research area and topic as well as expertise in the adopted methodology. In awarding a PhD, the examiners are also recognising you as an expert (if not the expert) on that particular topic. The viva is therefore best regarded as a discussion or debate between academics, one of them being the candidate. The examiners do not necessarily have to agree with the approach, argument, analysis or even outcome, provided you can adequately defend what you did, why you did it, and how you did it. Don't be afraid to ask for clarification if you fail to understand a line of questioning – this can provide useful thinking time.

Preparation for the viva

Successful performance depends not only on a good thesis or in-depth knowledge, but also on sound preparation. Supervisors will generally suggest a 'dry run' or rehearsal of the viva. If they do not, you might ask to be questioned in a formal or informal manner by supervisors and/or an outsider. Some universities or departments have public mock vivas (Delamont *et al.*, 1997) to indicate to candidates how their oral examination might be conducted. However, do be prepared for the examiners to pose completely different questions from those in the rehearsal.

Often, a number of months elapse between handing in the thesis and the viva. It is all the more important that you revisit the contents of the study by rereading it thoroughly shortly before the viva.

Example

One of us (Immy Holloway) had a period of more than nine months between submission and viva. She was too busy at work to reread the study thoroughly and make notes and therefore felt inadequate when asked about the location of some of her ideas in the thesis.

You might note down the location and page number of key concepts in each chapter and bring the notes to the viva. Another way of staying in touch with the thesis is the preparation of an article for publication or presentation of the findings at a conference.

Once you know the names of the examiners, you can find out whether you have referred to the expert examiner(s) in the thesis. It is essential that you understand the examiner's work before quoting and discussing it in the thesis as misrepresentation is probably a greater sin than omission. All examinees should, in any case, acquaint themselves with the examiner's ideas and ideology and avoid controversy or offence when discussing their own stance. It is only human for the examiners to be pleased when their work is known.

Examples

Mary had done her doctoral work on the socialisation of physiotherapists. Her external examiner was an eminent professor and an expert on socialisation processes of professionals. Mary had not mentioned his work in her thesis, in spite of her supervisor's advice. She did study his ideas as soon as she heard about his appointment and was able to discuss her thoughts on them at the viva. In the event, the external was satisfied with her work, even though he had clearly expected references to his own work in the thesis.

Roger, on the other hand, demonstrated in his thesis that he had misrepresented the external examiner's research and used concepts from it inappropriately. One of the reasons given for the failure was that the examiner felt that Roger's work was careless and lacked proper analysis and depth of understanding.

Some questions are typically asked in a viva, for example:

- Why did you choose this area (topic, problem) of study?
- What is the reason for your chosen research method (design, approach, methodology)?
- How did you know that participants answered your questions truthfully?
- Why did you not mention the seminal study of X in your research?
- Did you obtain any surprising results?
- What do you think is the most important contribution of your work to this field of study?
- How do your conclusions lead to the implications for practice?

Most of the questions that will be asked are more searching and specific, but it might boost your confidence if you are able to answer at least some of the above questions.

Recommendations

The recommendations on completion of the viva are similar for most institutions, although minor variations do exist. In most instances there are three main possibilities: a pass, a provisional pass or a failure. They might state, for instance, that:

(1) The award be made immediately.
(2) The award be made following some minor corrections (such as spelling errors and insubstantial flaws) which have to be amended as soon as possible.
(3) The candidate resubmit the thesis, subject to amendments, within an agreed time period (one or two years) for the approval of the examiners, with or without another viva.
(4) The candidate be given a lower award (such as an MPhil in the case of a PhD submission).
(5) The candidate resubmit to satisfy the examiners for an MPhil.
(6) The candidate fail outright without permission for re-examination

Exceptional cases

There are few circumstances when the candidate is exempt from the viva and these are stated by the UCoSDA (1995). This happens mainly for three reasons:

(1) When a well-known researcher submits a PhD by published research and the institutional regulations explicitly allow exemptions.
(2) When a candidate has an illness and would be seriously disadvantaged by the oral examination. This only happens in cases where the candidate's thesis is of a good enough standard to pass.
(3) When all examiners jointly agree that there is no point in a viva as the work is completely inadequate. In this case the externals would give written guidance to the student, as they do in other cases of failure.

Sometimes examiners decide before the viva that the written work is of sufficiently high quality to pass, but they would not generally let the candidate know this. In this case the viva provides an opportunity for the candidate to discuss the thesis, which, after all, represents the work of many years.

There has been a debate in the *Times Higher Education Supplement* recently, culminating in some interesting articles, some of which argued for the abolition of the viva. Gillon (1998) suggests that two main opposing camps exist. One argues for the retention of the traditional

PhD viva because this can demonstrate that the candidates have understood what they have written and not merely repeated what their supervisor suggested they say or repeated ideas from textbooks. The other camp believes that the viva situation is too pressurised and a number of factors may make it problematic: examiners are not generally acquainted with the candidates and all their other work; it is dangerous, too, that an important judgement relies on just one day of examining. This camp argues for a staged assessment of the PhD and for a new model to be developed. For students in health and social care, this would certainly be an advantage as academics in these fields believe in development and process rather than merely the product. Nevertheless, at the time of writing, the traditional PhD viva still exists and you will probably have to 'suffer' this.

The final, successful thesis will be available in the university library and on microfiche through the British Library.

The appeal process

While most individuals will probably never be in a position of going through an appeal, they might wish to learn about the appeal procedure in their university.

An appeal might be lodged if there is evidence that:

(1)   There has been an administrative error or the examination procedures were irregular.
(2)   Students have been ill or were adversely affected by factors not under their control (such as a death in the family).

Most examination appeals are made on the basis that the student has been unfairly treated and that inappropriate or unjust decisions have been made by examiners. Occasionally a student succeeds in overturning decisions of the examiners and achieves a review and re-evaluation of the thesis when it had failed. The student has to bring evidence that an injustice has been done, to a committee which includes independent members, and this is not easy. One main reason for failure is poor advice to the student to register for an MPhil or PhD in the first place, and poor supervision or supervisory contact during the period of registration. However, while these may give grounds for suing the university if the necessary evidence is provided, they do not provide sufficient reason to appeal against the outcome of the examination.

Common reasons for failure

The most common reasons for failure to complete or failing the examination include poor selection, poor supervision, mismatch between student, topic and/or supervisor and, particularly for part-time students, work overload, failure to prioritise successfully, and life interruptions and changes.

Poor selection

Selection involves both the student and the director of studies or first supervisor. We have offered advice to students on their selection of appropriate departments and supervisory teams. Supervisors are generally very careful in their selection of students. Nevertheless, mistakes can be made. You must be absolutely certain that you feel really enthusiastic about undertaking three years of full time study in the topic area proposed or a much longer time span as a part-timer. It is better to admit to doubts at the outset than be seduced into something that is manifestly wrong for all concerned. From the supervisor's perspective, it is essential to recruit only those students who have the necessary critical thinking skills and who are articulate on paper. A good first degree is probably the best indicator of this, and most universities demand this in any case.

Poor supervision

Poor supervisors fail to pay attention to the needs of their students, fail to read drafts of their work quickly and thoroughly, fail to provide their students with critical feedback (including praise), fail to pre-empt pitfalls, take on weak part-time students who do not have the requisite skills for study at this level and fail to counsel students when things start to go wrong. Poor supervision may be due to inexperience, *laissez-faire* attitudes, work overload or incompetence. You are advised to take responsibility for monitoring your own supervision and make sure that you are aware of formal and informal ways of addressing problems at an early stage. There are courses available nationally, if not internally, on research supervision. You are entitled to ask whether the supervisor has attended such a course and, if not, why not? This is particularly important if you know that your supervisor lacks experience, or if you have not had any opportunity to talk to other research students who have been supervised by the same supervisor.

Mismatch between student, topic and/or supervisor

We have dealt with most of these issues elsewhere. Don't be seduced into undertaking research for which you do not feel enthusiastic or fully committed. If you realise, after you have started, that you have made a mistake, discuss it with your supervisor or other mentor as soon as possible. It is better for all concerned to give up earlier than later.

Failure to prioritise

When writing the proposal for registration, you have to identify how much time you intend to devote to your research each week. Minimal expectations for part-time study are usually specified by the university, but it usually demands more, rather than less. Many students make unrealistic plans which they are unable to fulfil. It is necessary to sit down and work out how much time can reasonably be given at different stages of the research. It is advisable to see how much holiday and study leave can be accumulated to help with writing up as this is usually the most intensive period from the point of view of work and concentration. It is extremely difficult to complete the thesis if you have only the odd day here and there. It is also difficult to maintain the effort required to return to the literature review and bring all of the strands together with the findings.

A poor plan of research

Good supervisors should ensure that the original plan of research will answer the research question and be achievable within the time available. They will make certain that the research is rigorously planned and executed with an appropriate theoretical framework as well as valid and reliable methods of data collection and analysis. All of these aspects, together with the student's critical thinking and writing skills, should be tested at the stage of transfer from MPhil to PhD (see Chapter 8). At this stage, the supervisory team and research committee should give you critical feedback on the main strengths and weaknesses of the thesis. A good supervisor will counsel a weak student at this stage and may even recommend submission for an MPhil. If proceeding to a PhD, the good supervisor will ensure that the findings are subjected to systematic critical review, that the contribution of the thesis to the body of knowledge is clearly identified and articulated, that the aims of the research have been met and that the conclusions and recommendation for practice are fully supported by the findings and free of bias.

Example

John was a social work manager who chose to study the relationship between personality, stress and job satisfaction in staff working in residential care settings for the elderly. He hoped to demonstrate that some personality types were better suited to this type of work than others and felt that personality profiling may provide a useful recruitment tool. In his thesis, he had outlined theories of stress and coping and linked this to job satisfaction, citing research from other occupational groups. He asserted that personality was an important independent variable in the link between work demands and job satisfaction. He was advised by a local clinical psychologist to use a readily available measure of personality trait but, having no background in psychology, was unable to provide any direct theoretical link between the traits measured and adaptation to this type of work. In fact, this would have been difficult as personality trait theory and stress theory come from quite different schools of psychology. After a vast amount of data collection, he was able to identify only one personality trait which was significantly associated with low stress and high satisfaction, though difficult to interpret. Anecdotal evidence from informants suggested that situational factors may have been more important than personality, but no valid and reliable data, whether qualitative or quantitative, were available to support this. John wrote up his equivocal findings and presented them for examination. The thesis, though exceptionally well written and presented, failed to gain a PhD on the grounds that there was no real contribution to the body of knowledge in terms of theory (there was none), methodology (it was standard) or new facts (there were none). The examiner took the view that the thesis should be awarded an MPhil since it provided sufficient evidence of competence in the conduct and analysis of the research study.

John's problems should have been foreseen when his research proposal was scrutinised. The need to identify a suitable theoretical framework and measurement tools should have been identified (if not actually specified) at that stage. A broader literature search would have revealed that previous research into personality and occupation, cited in health care and psychology journals, had also

Contd.

drawn a blank. Expert advice from an academic psychologist specialising in stress would have warned against using a standard measure of personality trait because of difficulties in interpretation. A rigorous transfer process from MPhil to PhD would have exposed problems in the event of negative findings and John should have been advised to conduct another phase, using a rather more innovative methodology, to bolster his research and ensure its PhD-worthiness. Alternatively, John should have been advised of the possibility that the work would not achieve the criteria for PhD.

The anticlimax

Many students find that the period immediately after their viva seems like a dreadful anticlimax. Even if successful, the work which has pre-occupied them for so many years is suddenly history, leaving a large gap in their lives. Most students do not achieve an outright pass on the day of the viva but must make revisions of a minor or major nature. This inevitably delays the celebrations until the final thesis has been approved, by which time much of the excitement is lost. Furthermore, the timing of this may mean that the graduation ceremony can be up to a year later.

The real reward comes when you can legitimately put the letters after your name and, in the case of the PhD, call yourself 'Doctor'. (You will be amazed at the effect this title has in your private and public life. You might even get your car serviced more quickly!)

References

Burnham, P. (1994) Surviving the viva: unravelling the mystery of the PhD oral. *Journal of Graduate Education.* 1(1), 30–35.
Cryer, P. (1997) *Handling Common Dilemmas in Supervision.* Society for Research into Higher Education and the *Times Higher Education Supplement*, London.
Delamont, S., Atkinson, P. & Parry, O. (1997) *Supervising the PhD: a Guide to Success.* Society for Research into Higher Education & Open University Press, Buckingham.
Elton, L. & Members of the Task Force on Staff Development in Relation to Research (1994) Staff development in relation to research. In *Quality in Postgraduate Education* (eds O. Zuber-Skerrit & Y. Ryan), pp. 24–37. Kogan Page, London.

Gillon, E. (1998) A system in danger of overload. *Times Higher Education Supplement*, 15 May 1998.

Phillips, E.M. & Pugh, D.S. (1994) *How to Get a PhD: a Handbook for Students and their Supervisors*, 2nd edn. Open University Press, Buckingham.

UCosDA (1995) *Guidelines for Assessment of the PhD in Psychology and Related Disciplines*. British Psychological Society and the Universities' and Colleges' Staff Development Unit, Sheffield.

Further reading

National Postgraduate Committee (1995) *Guidelines for the Conduct of Research Degree Appeals*. Brandon House, Troon.

Partington, J., Brown, G. & Gordon, G. (1993) *Handbook for External Examiners in Higher Education*. Committee of Vice-Chancellors and Principals of the Universities of the United Kingdom, Universities Staff Development Unit, Sheffield.

Chapter 12

Disseminating the Research

Most researchers wish to place their work in the public arena for the scrutiny of peers. Having made a contribution to knowledge in a field or discipline, you will undoubtedly wish to disseminate it. Few theses reach a wide readership, and therefore the contents of the thesis needs to be published in some form so that the results are accessible and can be reviewed by peers. Indeed, if the work is not published, only the supervisors and examiners will ever read it.

You will be familiar with writing reports or assessments for your work. However, most health and social care professionals, with the exception of psychologists, do not come from a tradition of writing or publishing articles. Recently, however, more and more demands have been made on professionals to contribute to the literature which becomes publicly accessible information.

Occasionally a publisher might offer to publish your research in book form, and indeed a number of books are modified and adapted versions of theses (such as Melia, 1987; Lawler, 1991; Smith, 1992), although written journal articles are more common. In health and social care publication, it is important to communicate to the right audience so that improvements in treatment and care are shared and promoted. Indeed, Boyle (1997) suggests that one of the main reasons for publishing is to share knowledge. Even though the research may only increase the information about a topic area by a small amount or build on previous knowledge, sharing its findings and conclusions will gradually add to professional knowledge.

Reasons for publication

There are a variety of reasons why you might want to disseminate the research.

(1) You wish to familiarise the profession with the results of the work. No research is useful unless published in some form. Strauss and

Corbin (1998) assert that knowledge cannot accumulate if it is kept private and not made public.

(2) By writing or presenting papers at conferences, you can claim ownership of the particular research topic. If others are carrying out research in the same field, you demonstrate that you are well advanced and not merely replicating the work of others.

(3) Communication with peers may stimulate, start a valuable debate and advance the development of knowledge in the field.

(4) Publishing and presenting may enhance your career prospects. It is not only, as Boyle (1997) states, 'a prerequisite to success in an academic career' (p. 10), but it also enhances credibility in your discipline.

(5) Disseminating research will help to make you more confident, particularly when you present it at conferences.

(6) An article may challenge established beliefs and start a useful debate about an important issue.

Many supervisors suggest that students publish one or two interim papers for these and other reasons. Conference presentations are useful as critical reaction from other professionals helps to support, rationalise, modify or revise ideas. If supervisors are involved in advising you on your articles, or helping in writing them and contributing ideas, it is tradition and common courtesy to include their names in the published or publicised version. If research is carried out as part of a major project of a well-known academic in the field, it is essential to include the name of the professor. It is generally expected that anything published during the PhD process is seen and evaluated by the supervisor.

Choosing the readership and audience

When you present or write a research paper you usually address your peers unless the material is of great interest to the public. Sometimes you might present the material at professional conferences, but generally you might prefer sending the articles to the relevant and appropriate journals, about which supervisors and library will advise.

Journals may be professional or academic, depending on the tone and content of the article. A practically oriented article more often reaches a professional readership if published in a journal with a wide circulation (such as, for instance, the *British Medical Journal*, the *Nursing Times*, *Social Work Today*) while articles with a large element of theory can be found in academic journals (*Journal of Advanced Nursing, Sociology of Health and Illness, Journal of Social Work*). Supervisors will generally suggest an academic journal as it carries more status, and prestigious publications by PhD students in reputable, refereed journals help the university with its rating in the RAE. However, ultimately you yourself have to decide which journal would be appropriate, which readership you wish to inform and which type of articles will enhance your career. The best journals have referees who review the paper 'blind', that is, they do not receive the name or position of the writer when reading and evaluating it.

A good strategy for promoting one's work is to break it up into manageable chunks, for example the literature review, methodological or ethical considerations, and different aspects of findings. Start by submitting to present a conference paper or poster to gain some experience and critical feedback. Then prepare the article for submission to an academic peer-reviewed journal as these usually only wish to see work not yet published elsewhere. Allow at least six months for the process of refereeing and acceptance of revisions and a further year to 18 months to publication. Once accepted, prepare a summary report or overview for publication in a professional journal which will reach the widest readership. Occasionally, the editor will contact you if they have seen your original article in print.

Conference presentation

The number of conference presentations is usually limited because of the expense involved. Researchers generally choose just one or two of high prestige (such as the Medical Sociology Conference, the International RCN Conference, for instance). This guarantees an audience of peers. If you wish to present your research to date, you should submit an abstract to the organisers and hope it will be accepted. If so, the abstract for the paper will be printed in the conference abstracts and you will be informed about the presentation.

Taking an active part in a conference at a mid-stage in the research shows that you are able to claim ownership of the particular research topic. At the same time it prepares for the viva by giving you an opportunity to present your work in an open forum where questions can be asked. Levy (1996) gives useful guidelines for presenting a paper and stresses clarity of presentation and enthusiasm. He adds that the presenter should carefully plan and structure the material using appropriate audio and visual aids including a short handout.

The most difficult problem in presenting a conference paper is the management of time. Most conferences only allow for 15-minute presentations by delegates and five minutes for discussion. This means they cannot do full justice to the whole of a thesis. Crombie and Davies (1996) suggest that researchers limit their data and findings to the key points and reject material that is not directly related to the chosen focus. Jan Walker succeeded in presenting the bulk of her main findings during a ten-minute presentation at the World Congress on Pain. A set of about ten slides prepared using *Powerpoint*, or equivalent, ensures that only the most important information is conveyed. Another use of conference presentations was illustrated when one of Jan's students, having given a conference paper midway through her PhD studies, was approached by a well-known researcher who expressed an interest in being her external examiner. This often helps students' future careers.

Recently poster presentations have become more acceptable. The poster should be clearly presented visually, introduce the research, identify the methods and summarise the main findings and what they mean. The organisers will determine the size of the poster. Readers will not be interested in a crowded poster. Too many words obscure the information, while graphs and tables help give a clear picture. Printed summaries, including your e-mail address, on one side of A4 paper always go down well and may lead to future contacts. This is definitely a case of less is better. Set out merely to whet the appetite of passers-by and then spend your time chatting with them and exchanging names and addresses.

Writing a paper

Supervisors will often suggest that you write an article or two during the research process so that you get used to presenting your work in the public arena for scrutiny (this is not the custom at all universities). It is usual to write two or three papers (often with the main supervisor) on completion of a PhD. It is important that these articles differ from each other; at least they should have a different focus and be complete in themselves. The articles might include a literature review; reviews of key background, methodological, ethical or theoretical issues. This approach helps to ensure that you are able to publish several pieces of work from the research. Warren (1995), for instance, divided her MPhil research about the experience of hospital patients into three potential articles: one on the use of methodology; and two others based on findings. You must be aware, however, that 'salami slicing' a study for publication can also be detrimental as researchers often write too many articles which overlap in their contents about one single piece of research. Avoiding overlap and repetition is important.

The research paper should be appropriate for the journal to which it is sent and conform to its style, its way of referencing (generally Harvard or Vancouver), and its word limits. Before sending work to a journal, you might make sure you have seen the specifications and guidelines of the publisher, given, usually, on the first or last page of the journal. By reading some of the articles in the chosen journal and examining the general style and format, you have a better chance of your article being accepted by the editor of the journal. If in doubt, journals such as the *British Medical Journal* and *Journal of Nursing Management* have published extensive guidelines on writing for publication (these are available on application to the editor of the latter).

Example

A social worker encounters ethical problems during the pilot study of her research into children in care. These focus on differences in perception between social workers, families and the children themselves, and the need to respect and maintain confidentiality and privacy throughout. She writes up these dilemmas before embarking on the main study and finds that the feedback she receives, as a result of publication, from professional and academic colleagues very helpful.

Many of the guidelines for writing an academic essay can be applied to these types of article. An essay may contain a number of interesting elements and often several arguments as well as a discussion of well-known published work. A research article focuses on an important academic argument and/or a specific area of new knowledge in the field. Its length and type are determined by the guidelines set for the chosen journal.

Later articles based on the findings follow a structure similar to that of the thesis with an introduction, a method section, findings and discussion (in qualitative research findings and discussion can be integrated), as well as an overall conclusion, but the journal article is, of course, much shorter. The results of the paper will be compared with those of other published work. Readers expect writers to be truthful and accurate. All material submitted cannot be checked by the editor and referees of the chosen journal, or by a conference committee. Editors as well as readers are dependent on the writer's sense of responsibility as far as integrity and accuracy are concerned. Lack of integrity and inaccuracy of information in research papers can cause harm to patients and clients as well as destroy the reputation of researchers and their supervisors. Hall (1994) explains that authors must answer the following:

- What questions did you ask?
- How did you carry out the research?
- What did you find?
- What is the meaning of your findings?

The short introduction is aimed at setting the paper into context and gives the rationale for the research as well as its intentions. The research problem and the questions that have been addressed are defined as well as the reasons leading to these questions. Other writers' research papers, of direct relevance to the problem, need discussion as part of the background to the study. The methodology section provides a summary of the research design and strategies. The writer usually states how the problem has been treated in the research and which methodology was used. Depending on the journal, the methods used have to be described in great detail or can be short (for instance, the editors of many sociology journals would not expect a detailed discussion of grounded theory, a well-known research approach in the field, while nursing or midwifery journal editors require a more detailed description of methods). Unusual methods need a more detailed description. You should also describe any instruments and the statistical analysis used. Even in a 3000-word article you have to show how you carried out the design, sampling, data collection and analysis. A good paper includes the limitations of the strategies used. The article must demonstrate that ethical guidelines have been followed. The results section needs clarity, and the discussion should include the major findings, their significance and implications of the study for practice. The findings and their interpretation must be contextualised in relation to research of other writers. A short, succinct conclusion summarises what you have learnt in the course of the research.

Articles are always shorter and less explicit than theses, but they must be detailed enough for readers to understand both method and content. If you structure the writing logically, and if it has coherence, the paper is much more readable and more likely to be accepted. The findings are usually too long and complex to publish as a single article, and it is often better to divide them into two or three areas for submission to the same or different journals.

The article will rarely be accepted at the first attempt to publish. Journal editors either reject the paper outright or give conditional acceptance by suggesting that you change specific elements of the study. Rejection does not necessarily mean that the paper is irrelevant, but that it might not fit into the format or theme of the particular journal. Referees – generally independent experts in the field of health or social care – indicate where and how the article might be improved. The criticism should not be seen as a personal attack. You might not accept every aspect of the reviewer's critique, but you can use the critical comments to revisit the paper and change or refocus it. We have found in our own work that most articles improve on modification.

If acceptance of the paper is conditional, return it to the journal, as soon as possible after revision, taking critical comments into account. Write a covering letter in which you respond to the referees' comments point by point. For each, explain what modifications you have made to the text to address these, or the grounds on which you wish to take issue with the comments. Occasionally a journal will return a paper twice.

If the paper has been rejected, do not be deterred. If you feel that you can address the referees' comments, make the revisions and return with a covering letter, as above. We recently had an article rejected twice by a major international journal. The first time we made suitable revisions. The second time, we merely asked the editor to reconsider on the basis that the referee appeared to be biased against qualitative research. It was sent to another referee and accepted. Alternatively, you should address the referees' comments and send it to another journal in a revised version written specifically for the new journal. We have found that most articles will be published eventually if the writer has patience and is willing to revise the paper. To help you assess your own paper you might look at the following questions:

- Have I described the research question/problem? (WHAT)
- Have I described the setting and context? (WHERE)
- Did I mention the time frame of the research? (WHEN)

- Did I provide an adequate description of the sample and sampling method? (WHO)
- Did I justify the research? (WHY)
- Did I describe the research methodology and procedures? (HOW)

- What were the important findings of my research?
- What did I learn from my research?
- What are the implications for professional practice?

- Are my references complete and up to date?

- Have I followed *all* of the editor's guidelines?

Permission to publish

If you include the work of others in your research, you will of course attribute it to them and reference it. However, if you copy tables or diagrams or any other aspects of their research, you will need permission from the author or publisher. Academic publishers in the UK generally provide this permission as they have an agreement with each other, without asking the writer for financial compensation. However, US academic publishers and many commercial publishing firms in the UK and other countries charge for their permission to publish; and this charge will not be paid by the publisher of the journal or book. In many instances it is easier to use your own words to summarise the ideas of others and to reference the names of the original authors in the text.

You must consider the same ethical issues as those for the PhD. Anonymity of participants should be guaranteed and their confidentiality protected. In general the location should not be identifiable. If writing about an identified and identifiable location or organisation, you need permission to publish, in particular if you are carrying out funded research. The funding or grant-giving agency usually builds a clause into the contract to give it the right to deny permission to publish if, after scrutiny of the article, they disagree with its findings or conclusions. Do remember to send them copies of all publications or presentations before submission.

A word of warning. Some professionals are quite ready and willing to criticise their colleagues publicly in an article or a book. While there should not be any secrecy about mistakes or problems in health and social care settings which may emerge in the research, the reporting of these needs careful consideration. It is important to be truthful but advisable to be diplomatic and sensitive without attacking the actions or integrity of others.

References

Boyle, J. (1997) Writing it up: dissecting the dissertation. In *Completing a Qualitative Project*. (ed. J.M. Morse), pp. 9–37. Sage, Thousand Oaks, CA.

Crombie, I.K. & Davies, H.T.O. (1996) *Research in Health Care*. John Wiley & Sons, Chichester.

Hall, G.M. (1994) Structure of a scientific paper. In *How to Write a Paper* (ed. G.M. Hall), pp. 1–5. BMJ Publishing, London.

Lawler, J. (1991) *Behind the Screen: Nursing, Somology and the Problem of the Body*. Churchill Livingstone, Melbourne.

Levy, P. (1996) Presenting your research: reports and talks. In *Research Methods: Guidance for Postgraduates* (ed. T. Greenfield), pp. 253–268. Arnold, London.

Melia, K. (1987) *Learning and Working: the Occupational Socialisation of Nurses*. Tavistock, London.

Smith, P. (1992) *The Emotional Labour of Nursing*. Macmillan, Basingstoke.

Strauss, A. & Corbin, J.C. (1998) *Basics of Qualitative Research: Techniques and Procedures for Developing Grounded Theory*, 2nd edn. Sage, Thousand Oaks, CA.

Warren, J. (1995) *The Emotional Experience of People in Hospital*. Unpublished MPhil thesis, Bournemouth University.

Further reading

Becker, H.S. (1986) *Writing for Social Scientists: How to Start and Finish your Thesis, Book and Article*. University of Chicago Press, Chicago.

Cormack, D.F.S. (1994) *Writing for Health Care Professions*. Blackwell Science, Oxford.

Epilogue

Student and Supervisor Experiences

In this final chapter, we have included some examples of student and supervisor experiences to illustrate aspects which we think are significant. These are real examples. You will note that all of these reflect positive experiences. While we would have liked to present a contrasting experience, this would have necessitated so much modification to protect identities as to become little more than a work of fiction.

We have omitted the names of some institutions and individuals in the stories of experience.

The student experience: Jan Walker

I left health visiting to take a full-time degree in psychology. At the time I was finishing my degree, I saw a research assistant post advertised in my local higher education college (now a new university), with the opportunity to study for a PhD. The topic was 'pain in the community' and the supervisor was to be Dr (now Professor) Justus Akinsanya. I applied and was successful. Thus I found myself, in September 1986, with an empty office to myself and a research topic. The department was small and friendly and, although I was the only research student, I was made to feel at home amid colleagues from a variety of academic (sociology, biological sciences) and professional (nursing and social work) backgrounds, most of whom were studying for higher degrees on a part-time basis. Justus and I agreed a second supervisor of my choice, a psychologist from my previous university. Together, we set about negotiating the bureaucratic hurdles of the then Council for National Academic Awards (CNAA) who had responsibility for my registration, progress and ultimate award.

My first task was to write the research proposal. I had no idea what this might look like, quite apart from the fact that I had little detailed knowledge of research methodologies. My first attempt was sent back by the CNAA committee on three grounds, one of which was that I had failed to justify why I had assumed that rheumatoid arthritis was a painful condition! They also required the inclusion of another nurse academic on my supervisory team.

There were research students in the college at that time and the research training programme was severely limited. Nevertheless, my colleagues were generous with advice in terms of theoretical backgrounds (including systems theory which I still don't understand) and methodologies. I started reading and realised that, if I was to make progress, I would need a word processor. The department kindly obliged. I opted to use quantitative methods, since I already had a reasonable grounding in statistics, and set about establishing a theoretical framework. I started to develop ideas of my own about the nature of pain experience and requested weekly sessions with Justus to brainstorm these ideas. The best advice he ever gave me was to put these ideas into the form of a diagram or flow chart. This I put onto a white board in my office and tested it out on passers-by. It enabled me to distinguish dependent from independent variables and I then set about identifying suitable measures. One of the most difficult problems I faced was the tension between using existing psychological measures of quality of life, stress, depression, etc. which were valid and reliable and allowed comparability with other research, and the ethics of asking large numbers of intrusive questions. I opted to develop short and simple measures, thus ensuring that my work would not be deemed publishable in psychological journals. Fortunately, nursing journals were more forgiving.

My three years of study were wonderfully enjoyable. This was largely due to my regular dose of enthusiasm and motivation from Justus, and reassurance and encouragement from my second supervisor. My other supervisor had a rather different theoretical stance, and although I now see that he was actually quite right in many of his observations, it was not apparent to me at the time. I had been advised that doing a PhD would have its highs and lows. I had a brief low when a group of nurses who had pledged their support refused to complete a set of questionnaires concerning patients I had already interviewed. However, all researchers must learn sooner or later that, when the chips are down, they are the only ones who are fully committed to their research. My lowest ebb was when I ran my first multiple regression analysis and gained an answer that I had not expected. However, a few days later I negotiated a stronger regression model which proved to be more exciting than I had envisioned and all was back on track. I encountered a problem towards the end of my second year when I realised that local authority funding would not (as I had been led to believe) extend to a third year. I wrote hundreds of begging letters to a variety of organisations and received £50 from Lloyds Bank. I don't recommend this strategy! Justus eventually used his network of contacts to help me win a studentship from the Department of Health for one year.

The only disagreement I ever had with Justus was towards the end of writing up. I had presented and discussed my results and reached what I thought was a reasonable theoretical conclusion. Justus pointed out that a PhD in nursing must include a final chapter on the implications for nursing. I was tired and angry but, of course, he was absolutely right. I set about rounding off my thesis in a more sensible way and handed it in three years from the day I first started. I had three external examiners representing nursing, gerontology and health psychology. Fortunately, two examiners were satisfied and one required only fairly minor modifications. Although I would never subject my own students to this level of scrutiny, I have remained in close contact with one examiner and have recently re-established useful contact with another.

Justus insisted that I start writing for publication from an early stage and I had three articles in print, plus a review in the *Nursing Times*, before my study was completed. I was awarded £200 towards the cost of attending the World Congress on Pain in Hamburg by an educational trust at my training hospital (Barts). Justus introduced me to James Smith, editor of the *Journal of Advanced Nursing*, who, in turn, provided me with other important contacts. With encouragement from my supervisors, I presented my work at various national and European conferences in nursing and psychology, culminating in an oral presentation at the World Congress on Pain in Adelaide in 1990.

As I write this, I feel a glow of excitement and pride as I realise just how fortunate I was during those three years. Looking back, there were huge elements of luck: being given such an interesting topic to research; having such excellent supervisors; and finding myself so well supported in a small department and college. I loved every minute of it and am now trying to ensure that my own research students have an equally good experience.

The student experience: Marie Mills

After about a year in residential care work, and with no first degree, I thought I would like to know more about older people. Twelve years later, still with no first degree, I began my PhD studies as a part-time student, and completed in three years. This is not to say that I studied intensively during the preceding years. Rather, I meandered through various courses related to residential care of the elderly. Obtaining the Certificate in Social Services (CSS) (now subsumed into the Diploma in Social Work) was my highest ambition. At this time I was working in the private sector, and there was no large parent organisation to fund me. However, I besieged national charities who were very generous and paid my tuition fees, probably because at that time so few people from the independent sector were professionally qualified.

One of the courses was a post-qualifying course in ageing, health and social work at an established university. It was run by Dr (now Professor) Peter Coleman, an internationally renowned psychogerontologist. After this, I was persuaded by an organisation for whom I did some part-time work to do a research diploma in aspects of elderly care. I went for the initial interview at the polytechnic (now a university) nearby with some trepidation. I had very little understanding about 'proper' research and no knowledge at all about methods, analysis and statistics. Frankly, they seemed rather nasty to me and certainly had most preposterous names: 'grounded theory', 'Spearman rank correlation coefficient' and so on. I was honest about my ignorance, the interview went well, and I was accepted. From the start I was drawn to qualitative methods and, in fact, ended up using grounded theory in my study of the use of reminiscence and counselling in dementia. Even so, I remember being determined to have some understanding of quantitative methods and read a particularly dense and weighty tome one weekend. This was to confirm my dislike of 'number crunching' for another few years.

However, I found I really enjoyed the research process. I liked meeting the participants, their relatives and care staff. I found unexpected satisfaction in piecing information together, looking at the world in unfamiliar ways and learning how to recognise and analyse patterns of behaviour. I also thought it exciting to find theories that explained and supported observed phenomena. Through regular weekly interviews, I found my developing relationships with the participants to be very rewarding and surprisingly close.

The study was to produce three published papers, two in very respectable journals and the third was reprinted in a book. Using the investigation as a pilot, I decided to undertake a larger study and applied to the social work department where I had studied previously. As a mature student, my initial research studies allowed me access to the postgraduate programme. The reasons for choosing this particular university were quite pragmatic. Firstly, it was fairly close to my home, and it was also a course recognised and funded by the Central Council for Education and Training in Social Work (CCETSW). Finally, and most importantly, it would be supervised by Peter Coleman. I have since realised how fortunate I was to have him as a supervisor, and how important it is to choose one's supervisor with as much care as the research topic. The PhD process is after all a minimum of three years and benefits from positive relationships. Certainly, to have respect and liking for the person guiding your path through the intricate maze of research and university procedures makes life much easier. Moreover, a supervisor acting as a mentor can have great influence on future career prospects.

During my informal interview, I was asked why I wanted to do a PhD, and the reasons were many. Some seemed quite frivolous – I quite liked the idea of my family calling me 'Doctor'. Others were more serious – unlike some older people in care, I did not want to enter my own old age with regrets about underachievement, of not making the most of my mind. I was also aware that I wanted to know more about my tripartite area of interest, the role of emotions in memory and dementia.

In due course I was offered a funded part-time place on the MPhil/PhD programme. I wasn't sure what to do at first, and although there were a series of lectures to attend, they were basically similar to those given at my previous institution. My second supervisor, who was also a psychologist, had dismissed my initial fears of knowing nothing about psychology, saying it was a very imprecise science, and the job of a university was to teach students to teach themselves. I decided 'to teach myself' and began by avoiding the lectures and spending the time in the library researching the literature. At that time, little was written about emotion and dementia, although Tom Kitwood's 'new culture of dementia care' was beginning to make a great impact and paved the way for more qualitative psychological investigations into dementia. There were also few longitudinal studies on this topic.

My own study eventually consisted of case studies of eight older people with dementia whom I saw over a two-year period. Data consisted of over 140 recorded and transcribed interviews, resulting in nearly 800 pages of text. I tended to try and transcribe the interviews as soon as possible after the interview, often on the same day. I was quite anxious about doing this as soon as I could, perhaps feeling that I could become overwhelmed if interviews were left to pile up, although I was fortunate in having good audio typing equipment due to an award made by the Social Work Educational Trust. I recall many months of trying to organise a sea of paper, reading the literature, frequent visits to the setting and Friday afternoon tutorials, plus, of course, working three days a week. It was a heady and delightfully enjoyable time.

However, there were some bad patches. I was refused permission to include participants' case studies in the main body of the thesis, although they were allowed to be part of the appendices. As these case studies largely consisted of their own words, this decision felt like a rejection of their contributions. Having completed the thesis, I was then required to write another chapter on the findings, subjecting them to second-order analysis. I was also very nervous about the viva and found it hard going. My external assessor requested that some changes be made, and I felt quite angry about this as I did not want to expand my work in the direction he suggested. In addition, there was an extremely civilised lunch for the four of us afterwards, although I did not feel very civilised and would rather have liked to have had a tantrum. I felt very tired. However, I had to admit that the changes, which were completed in a week, greatly strengthened my argument, and I have often been grateful for the external's intervention. He has commented on my work favourably over the years and recommended me to others.

Graduating is also part of the PhD process, and I remember my graduation with much pleasure. It was a beautiful day and the campus was covered in marquees overflowing with students and staff in amazingly varied and colourful academic robes. My family were there, together with Peter Coleman and another tutor from my CSS days. It was a great time, followed by other equally enjoyable celebrations. I was fortunate in being asked to present my findings in Amsterdam at the Third European Congress of Gerontology later that year, and to take part in a European symposium on therapeutic work with older people at the University of Stirling. I have also spoken about my work at other seminars and conferences, published a number of papers and turned my thesis into a book.

As I look back I recall why I wanted to do a PhD and, yes, I do think I know more than I did before. Not only about my own area of interest, but also about other subjects gleaned from fellow students and the academic world in general. I feel I have achieved, although this is not as important as it once was, and there are still many things I would like to learn. However, it is probable that no other learning situation will ever match my PhD years. I think of them as providing a highly exhilarating roller coaster of a journey which gave me one of the most significant and intense experiences of my life. Would I recommend this journey to others? Without any hesitation. It is a time when the key to endless possibilities is given to you.

The supervisor experience: Justus Akinsanya

When I arrived [at an institute of higher education] in 1985, nursing and social work courses were well established in the institution. Applied research was a strong aspect of the nursing courses and my predecessor had established a strong link with the local hospitals. My previous post had a strong research component and I was resolved to establish a credible research profile in my new post, which meant giving preference to research activities. The directorate supported and encouraged me. It was necessary to have the support of departmental staff, and the head led by example. We agreed that my priority was to establish the research credibility of the department.

I was anxious to start a postgraduate programme in the department and the Department of Health and Social Security (DHSS) included it on the national annual list of centres eligible for research awards. The director of the institute was encouraged by this recognition and decided to support the department to employ a research assistant to undertake a funded study for an MPhil/PhD. The choice of topic was left open and I chose to focus on the management of pain – my former supervisor Professor Jack Hayward had researched the area and was a visiting professor to the institute. I wrote a draft proposal based on my wife's article on the topic of pain in the community which was published in *Nurse Education Today*. The proposal was approved for funding for two years and, if a successful MPhil transfer stage was reached, the department was expected to seek external funding for the PhD stage. We placed advertisements in the press and waited to see who would apply. Many enquiries were received by telephone, letters and in person. One of the enquiries was from Jan Walker, who was due to graduate in psychology from a nearby university. I invited her for an informal visit and was immediately impressed by her academic, professional and personal particulars. She successfully applied for the post of research assistant to undertake a two-year study and to be registered for the MPhil/PhD degree.

Jan was provided with an empty office and was advised to request supplies. I was absolutely delighted when I found that she was able to touch type and use a computer. She was provided with a computer for personal use and immediately settled down to work. She astonished me by being so quick, efficient and accurate in the preparation of her application to register for the MPhil/PhD. The proposal was submitted to the research degrees committee, approved and recommended for submission. The application was forwarded to the CNAA and after amendments – relating to the supervisory team and theoretical aspects – it was accepted. Jan was duly registered with three members in her supervisory team. The bureaucratic procedure of the CNAA for registration had to be followed to the letter. Indeed, looking back now, I am sure that it was right and essential to do so as a learning experience for individuals who might not have had the experience of supervision at that level. I certainly had no previous supervisory experience of doctoral students and was most anxious to learn.

My relationship with Jan was perfect. We got on famously throughout the three years. I was made a reader and head of the enterprise and research unit; then promoted to a personal chair in nursing. Jan was my first doctoral student and I was determined that she would get every support, as I had from Professor Jack Hayward. Supervision is a crucial undertaking for all concerned, especially for the student. It is the student who has to do the work and it helps if all those around the student provide encouragement, support and understanding. As a supervisor, I learned not to interfere with my student's research stance but to offer abundant support and encouragement. As Jan rightly put it, I've learned to accept the fact that the student's ownership of the qualification is best safeguarded during supervision. After all, it is the student's work and one to be proud of in the future. In any event, Jan's work was based on psychology and although this was a subject I'd studied as part of my own human biology degree, I could not understand the level that Jan had taken it to. We had two psychologists as additional supervisors and I relied on them for disciplinary guidance.

It is now over a decade since Jan completed her PhD, and looking at my copy of the thesis again while preparing this contribution has brought back happy memories: the unpredictable changes and the various stages involved; the patience and commitment; the institutional and departmental support and, above all, the fact that it all ended successfully. I feel proud and privileged to have had such a first supervisory experience. It has to be admitted that we were lucky but above all we had mutual respect for each other. On my part, I have to say that I admired Jan for her incisiveness, intellectual ability and readiness to engage in debate. I believe that these are essential research qualities at the MPhil/PhD level.

Further reading

Salmon, P. (1992) *Achieving a PhD: Ten Students' Experiences*. Trentham Books, Stoke-on-Trent.

Index

abstract of research proposal 89
  structure 135–6
Academic Quality and Standards, code of
  practice 110
acknowledgements (thesis) 136–7
aim statement 139
Alzheimer Disease Society 31
American Psychological Association,
  PsycLIT abstracts 77
appeals procedure 159
appendices 145–6
applied research, defined 3
article for publication *see* research paper
Association of Medical Charities 31
attribution, permission to publish 172–3
authorship, false attribution 129

Bath Information and Data Services
  (BIDS) 77
Beauchamp-Childress, ethical behaviour
  principles 57–8
beneficence, defined 63
bibliography, maintenance 73–4
Biotechnology and Biological Science
  Research Council (BBSRC) 30
British Library 77
British Medical Journal (BMJ), guidelines
  for writers 169
British Psychological Society (BPS) 22
  examination criteria 152

Care data, database 76
Central Council for Education and
  Training in Social Work (CCETSW)
  30–31
charities, Association of Medical Charities
  31
Citation Index for Nursing and Allied
  Health (CINAHL) 76
closed circuit television (CCTV), ethical
  issues 61
Cochrane and York databases 77
Code of Practice for the Assurance of
  Academic Quality and Standards 110
completion rates, part-time students 19
conclusion (thesis) 144–5

conference presentation of research paper
  167–8
confidentiality *see also* ethical issues
confidentiality agreement 58
confidentiality practice 58–9
  example 59
  referral necessity 61
  vulnerable groups 59
consent to research 59–60, 66–7
  basic components 65
  form and reply templates 66–7
creativity concept 10–11
critique, defined 74

data, falsification 129
data analysis 142
data collection 142
Declaration of Helsinki (1964 rev. 1975) 57
degree committee, research proposal,
  criteria 87
design of research 90–91
  timetable 97–9
discussion (thesis) 144
dissertation *see* thesis
Doctor of Business Administration (DBA)
  14–15
Doctor in Clinical Psychology
  (DClinPsychol) 14–15
Doctor of Education (DEd) 14–15
Doctor of Medical Science (DMedSci)
  14–15
duplication of research by others 127–8

e-mail, inter-university 78
Economic and Social Research Council
  (ESRC) 30
enrolment, defined 32
enrolment preparation 17–32
  educational prerequisites 17–20
  highly specialised equipment/expertise
  24
  location of topic 20–22
  paying own fees, issues arising 23–4
  peer experiences 25–6
  PhD joint subject supervision 23
  university/department selection 23–4